WRITING ON MY PILLOW

WRITING ON MY PILLOW

A Memoir of Generational Change
and an Acupuncturist's Climb
Out of Addiction

ROBIN RAE ROEMER

Board Certified Acupuncturist Oriental Medicine

Writing On My Pillow: *A Memoir of Generational Change and an Acupuncturist's Climb Out of Addiction*

Copyright © 2021, Robin Rae Roemer

Library of Congress Control Number: 2021915763

ISBN: 979-8-53716654-2

Printed and bound in the United States of America

FIRST EDITION

October 8, 1980, was the day I signed up with my Creator,
to begin and stay sober, clean, and clear. First and foremost,
I dedicate this book to my Creator, the anniversary of my rebirth,
and my son Trever Dylan Brown who is deeply connected to
my motivation to write this book.

Fasten your belts it's a dysfunctional ride

Inbred, ingrained, logged in, no way out, looking for a guide

Accept twelve steps endured until embodied,

forever changed, God and I allied

Now in compassion for the results of that pain only to divide

Reappear in different shapes, sizes, times, truly patient and wide

Dysfunction rears its ugly head unexpected,

surprise, start again, crucified

Have faith, Jesus did, don't give up,

the truth will abide

Table of Contents

Acknowledgments

Thank you to my Creator, all my spiritual guides, religious leaders, spiritual practitioners, teachers, guides, family, friends, outside help, sponsor's and sponsee's who are here and who have come and gone. I would not be able to write this book without the dysfunctional events from my family trauma. I have compassion and forgiveness and I'm truly blessed by your presence.

I would like to thank my father for passing away sober, steadfastness, reliability, teaching me a strong work ethic. My mother for teaching me thoughts are things, the power of the mind, "There is a Way" no matter the obstacle, an answer will come. For sending me notes of love in the mail and reminders my whole life. Both of my parents for showing their confidence in me by being a long-time alternative medicine and acupuncture clients of mine since 1992. My ex-husband for his allowing me the space to write this book. My son for the strong leading spirit he is. Both physically, mentally and spiritually supporting me during the times of my nuclear family crisis.

My stepdaughters for all they have taught me.

Preface

After experiencing a deeply profound and transformational healing session a few years ago, through power, wisdom, and goodness, I became aware that I signed up for my role in this life— to break something generational; being raised by perpetrators in alcoholism, emotional abuse, rejection, betrayal, materialism, and conditional love, using drugs and alcohol. At the time, I thought, *Wow, why would I do that? That's quite a painful assignment.* More clarity has come since then, and I know—*without a doubt*—that I was brought here through my mother by my Creator to learn life's lessons so that I could teach others about their lessons. I am here to bring joy, inspiration, faith, and love to those who may not otherwise see, hear or feel this truth.

"Who would ask for that?" you might ask, in disbelief. *I would.* My soul signed up to experience an adventure. I was born with the ability to experience major extremes, so that I could learn from the contrast, grow emotionally, mentally, and spiritually from my healing, and have clarity and certainty about what I value in life, and learn how to love myself in a positive way. As I reflect on the

mountains, I climbed to gain this clarity, the courage and fortitude I developed were what finally allowed me to see that *I could actually climb over and out.*

I used to write a lot as a child. Nothing happens until I write. The dream, the goal, the desire. My name, the date, my aspiration. I, Robin Roemer Brown, am giving this book as an offering of trust, inspiration, guidance, and light to others suffering from addiction, or those affected by dysfunction or self-sabotage of any type. This was inspired by my mother, my life experience, and a quote

"I learned that courage was not the absence of fear, but the triumph over it. The brave man is not he who does not feel afraid, but he who conquers that fear." -Nelson Mandela

My way reveals itself to the degree that I am willing and wanting to move my perspective. I've had to learn how to get out of my own way and remove my self-imposed shackles so many times that I can't possibly count. The most recent of which was in the middle of finishing this book. I am either the problem or the answer, depending upon my outlook and the frequency I am tuned to. I call it a boomerang.

Different from a recovery process, *Writing on My Pillow* is written with a broader brushstroke for a larger audience than just the addicted, afflicted, or recovering. Its principles can be used to bring peace to anyone who feels ill-at-ease in their skin and in the world. It's words are written, not only with the intention to bring hope and inspiration, but also to offer methods that can be applied to any dilemma, for any individual, and in any given moment, to achieve immediate relief and lasting results.

I wrote these pages for you, no matter who you are, or what you have gone through, or how easy or horrible your life may be, or if it is an addiction, depression, fear, self-denigration, financial or relationship loss, or health challenge that has or had you in its grip. It may not even be you. You may be connected with someone who has experienced a rough patch, or a life patch or is currently in one, spiraling downward. No matter who, what, how, when, or why, my words are to help you. As one who has come out the other side and blossomed in spite of it, *and because of it,* I have written this book to show how to handle the inner demons and balance the conflicting energies that seem to overpower you.

Written in two parts, Part I details my entrance and deepening into the adversity that was the first twenty-two years of my life experience. It is told from the energy I was in at the time and the perspectives I had of myself, my family, and my world. When you're in it, you cannot see your part, and you cannot see a way out. Part II describes my way out, the changes in myself, my family, and my world, the resources I used to design my new life, and what I teach others to help them design their new lives.

It is my hope that my story and profound spiritual change can be a lamplight, illuminating the world you see yourself in, and helping to light your way to a better life.

– Blessings, Dr. Robin

Introduction

A severe limitation came into my life at a very young age. Through a severely oppressive and depressive environment, I was stifled and stunted emotionally, mentally, and physically. Without the freedom and permission to express my feelings, thoughts, and desires, I had to conform to the environment to survive.

Because the diseases of alcoholism and narcissism are ones in which every family member is adversely affected in some way, individual denial is enormous. Each member is blinded, believing they do not have a problem, which creates a need for self-preservation and keeps the individuals addicted to the behavior of denial, codependency, and abuse, or to the addiction of drinking, or both. Each blames one or more of the others and denies responsibility for their part. The family typically adapts to the chemically dependent person, or persons, by taking on roles that help reduce the individual or environmental stress, deal with uncertainty, and allow the family to function within the craziness and fear that is created by the addict.

Being born into and raised in a disease-addicted environment inherently resulted in my feeling of being treated as if I had five parents: Mom, Dad, older sister, older brother, older sister. Never validated. Continually being told what to do—*often by more than one relative in a given situation*—stamped me as the family scapegoat. The scapegoat is often very successful at distracting the family and others from the addicted individual. Forced to conform to the disease-induced dysfunction during my early childhood development, I learned to adapt by stirring up trouble or concerns, to deflect attention away from the real issue, *which, in my case, was my dad.* I was indoctrinated from birth into adulthood with this condition and its lessons—and the shame inflicted with it.

My energy slowly declined, and my development in all areas became both distorted and repressed.

But this is not that story. This is not a story of tragic endings. This is a story of renewal and inspiration. This is a story of healing, triumphs of the human spirit, and transformation.

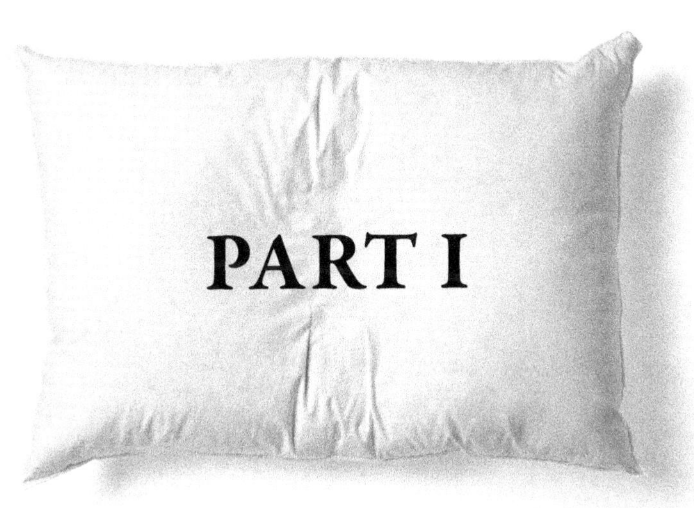

PART I

CHAPTER 1

Perpendicular Love

Mother told me that she had to hold herself up on the table for hours, so as not to crush me. When the huge surge of energy hit her, she was more than ready, and out I finally came into the world. *"Robin Rae Roemer should be the stage name of an actress, or someone famous; it has such a great rhythm,"* she used to say.

As the youngest child of four children, I was a ball of energy with no room to bounce. I shared a room with my brother until I was four. The youngest of my older sisters was very needy and required a lot of attention. I was two or three when she was diagnosed with strabismus. Her eyes didn't look in the same direction at the same time, so she had to do eye exercises every day for a year. On most mornings, I toddled my way behind her and my mom through the house, out the laundry room, into the back yard, and to the garage, to sit on the back porch while Mom helped her do exercises to stop her roving eye. I was happy that the muscles eventually strengthened to hold her eye straight and that she didn't need eye surgery, but having this responsibility for a whole year seemed like a long time to a fidgety me.

She needed help with other things too. Her foot was turned at an angle, facing the wrong way. And she needed attention for her knee that turned inward. Then there was the night she swallowed a chicken bone and almost choked to death at dinner. And there was that serious melanoma cancer scare that was one millimeter close to entering her lymphatic system. To this day, a rather large scar remains on her shoulder.

Ours was an intellectual home, not a soft, huggee, kissy, or lovey home. My parents were always busy, sick, or asleep. Watching TV which was busy. Reading the paper was busy. Drinking was busy. Affection was rarely shown. *"Of course, we love you,"* my mom said. Personally, I did not feel the emotion in any of their spoken words. I was full of energy and sensitive to energy, so I was regularly shut down, ignored, or overwhelmed. I ran away when I was four years old. My mom laughed at me, telling me I had nowhere else to go.

I did not know what to do with my feelings, so I began writing on my pillow, nestled in the only safe space I knew, the corner of my bed. If something harmed or scared me, I could express my feelings only on my pillow, hoping God would listen.

Around four and a half, I moved into my younger older sister's room. As an active, always moving child, my mom began tying my sheets tightly to the bed with clips at night so I wouldn't kick my covers off and get cold or sick. I woke my sister up with my thrashing about the room. I needed to engage and feel connected and close, but she liked to read books and be disengaged. So, she hid out by herself to read. When I tried to talk to her, she got mad. I was also not as orderly and private as she was. She got so upset one time that she drew a line on the floor across the entire room and said, *"This is your side, and this is mine."*

When we moved into our new house in Stratford Square, Long Beach in 1961, my sister got the first choice on which bunk she wanted on our new bed. The next day, while bouncing up and down on my bunk, I jumped too high, landing too close to the outside edge and fell on the floor on my neck. My parents were busy, so I got up and said I was ok. They were on a very tight budget and didn't have extra money, and mom was raised Christian Science. So, unless one of us had a respiratory illness or a temperature above one hundred and three, there were no doctor visits. No one paid attention to my fall, so I forgot all about it.

From a young age, I did not feel safe. My room was filled with conflict from my youngest older sister. I often felt hurt and uncomfortable and continually sought approval from my mom. On the rare occasions when she read to me at night, I was soothed by her voice. The rest of the time, I could only count on my Kewpie doll. He smiled at me and glowed. My mom had opened him up and put a pink heart in him. He was the only thing I didn't have to share with anyone and helped me to feel secure in my bed in my little corner.

My youngest older sister was the first to get what she needed. When my mom had two of something, my sister chose first. If I needed something, I had to wait until she was attended to. There was never enough money, and I got hand-me-downs and whatever was left. I assumed that I wasn't good enough to receive the things I needed or new things and that she was more important than I. If I was having trouble or slow to get something, she rushed to tell my parents. At first, I thought she cared, but after a while, I began to see that she had a self-serving agenda, a goal that included one-upmanship. Forever in a ploy for attention, she had no regard for me, and only complained about me.

Age 7 in second-grade class I was acting out, challenging my teacher, I made some comments and acted as a class clown a few times. I felt I was witty. I was trying to be funny. Well, in second grade, my teacher told me I had to take my desk and sit in the hallway and then she put a Dunce Hat on me. I had to wear it. Well, I told no one for quite a while, because the way I felt I was somewhat similar treated at home I felt the experience was not much different. I never knew whether support was coming or whether I was going to be verbally cut like a knife. My best ongoing daily example was dismissing and belittling behavior (often presented as humor), In other words, Emotionally unsafe.... And the punishment not fitting the crime. I did not want to get into trouble at home because of school discipline so I told no one for quite a while. Dad was traveling for work and was not home for a week or two at a time during that time of my life. After one month the principal of the school called my mom and mom did come to my rescue. I felt happy she did. She told me after speaking with the Principal, the teacher did not possess the skills to handle me. She said I would have a fantastic teacher in the third grade. At 7 years old I felt that was a long time away and the damage was done.

By third grade, I could not read or comprehend what I did read, so I was required to be evaluated for "my problem" and I needed outside reading classes. I felt very stupid now. Not realizing the emotional trauma had something to do with my confidence. Being a great swimmer helped me feel better about myself, and I swam with my sister's class of twelve-year old's. The coach wanted to train me for Olympic swimming, but my mom said no. My heart sank. I was more than disappointed. In addition, my sister began telling me things like, *"You're not smart. You're not smart enough yet. You will never make that,"* and other putdowns, like, *"You're too young to know about that. You're not invited. You're not wanted here."* Living in the same room for years with my youngest older sister stepping on me and knocking me around verbally and mentally, I lost my self-confidence little by little, as well as my sense of safety, ability to be happy, and belief that I was lovable. The severity of her needs continually took precedence, displacing me and my needs. She had to win all arguments and excelled in explaining her way to the top, or to the place where she appeared right. Internally, I learned to just give in. The negative analytical energy was too draining and consuming for me, not worth constant fighting. As the years went by, I understood that she needed more attention than I.

My parents paid the most attention to me when I was sick. Somehow, I managed to have tonsillitis every other month. Being a sensitive child in my dysfunctional family environment contributed to my increasing insecurity. At some point, the knowledge that I had not been wanted, was not invited, was not a part of the family had solidified in my psyche. I heard these types of references regularly from my younger older sister in the privacy of our bedroom, but I could not identify the initial source or specific time I had heard it. I felt adopted, despite my mom telling me, *"Honey we love you, and you are not adopted."*

After sharing a room with my sister for many years, I grew tired of her cruelty and began to recognize that she was just trying to manipulate me with her gaslighting, continual criticism, asserting dominance by making it difficult for me to make decisions or punishing me when I did. This gaslighting, smothering behavior that attempts to control or keep tabs on me and attempting to isolate me by driving a wedge between me and my support system. These are all abusive tactics. I realized that I needed to develop tools to stand up for myself. By incessantly watching my family members interact, debate, argue with one upmanship tactics daily. I learned about power and how one could use it against another. I learned from monkey see monkey do how to tap into a person's internal operating system and use it against them. I learned how I could negotiate, con and mentally stab and trick from a power place. I found these tools necessary for my survival, and I used them more and more to help defend myself and get what I needed.

My dad traveled a lot, early on when I was a baby, so I don't recall having him around much, except one memory. I was three to four, sitting on his lap while he gave me sips of his Pabst Blue-Ribbon beer. When I was older, and he was home more, I was always excited to show him what I had learned that day. I'd do each round-off or cartwheel ten times as I learned them. Ninety-five percent of the time, he'd arrive home between five fifty and six o' five. I was amazed by his ability to do that. If he was going to be late, he'd call to let us know. This created a feeling of stability and security. I could always count on his consistency.

Money was very high up on my parents' list of values. My Dad pointed out to us anyone who had money. We never had enough. He'd let us sit on the roof and watch the fireworks, or sneak us into Veteran's Stadium to watch. I found out later he couldn't afford to buy tickets for everyone. He followed fire trucks to the fires. I was never sure what he was doing, but he always had a reason. Maybe he was fascinated with fire.

A chronic teaser with a dry sense of humor, Dad was always ready with a smart-aleck innuendo that bordered on bullying. Although there was great humor in our house, and my parents generally talked and decided important issues together, we were raised in a variation of tyranny. He'd frequently raise his hand to give the famous Hitler Sieg Heil salute. I'd look at him, puzzled. He called himself a dictator, seeing himself in charge. He expressed himself more powerfully by telling us, *"I am the chief, and don't you forget it."* He often commented, *"There are too many chiefs and not enough Indians,"* or *"Children should be seen and not heard,"* or *"Shut those brats up"* A master of rules, he was prone to sarcastic rage, often using his voice to invoke shame throughout the house. Somehow, though, he managed to remain calm while doing this.

In general, the holidays were more fun for me, visiting our relatives' homes and having them at ours. Mom was always busy, so if

I needed help on some task, she'd delegate it to one of my older siblings. The exception was the night before Christmas, which was one of the few times we had special alone time.

On Christmas morning, I woke up at six-thirty and bounced around my room in anticipation of eight o'clock. Then the four of us were allowed to come out of our rooms and line up behind the closed hallway door. At eight-ten, the hallway door opened, and we'd rush over to the fireplace to open our stockings. We were permitted to do this on our own. Afterward, my siblings took the presents out from under the tree and distributed them to each of us. I usually sat on the brown couch next to my dad in his chair, and my mom sat in her chair. We were not allowed to have any drinks or food, because we might spill on the table. We had to wait for everyone to receive their gifts before we could begin opening them, and someone always had to go to the bathroom at the last minute.

Most of the time, my dad received the most gifts, because of his business vendors and others who loved him. My favorite of his gifts was See's candy. We got to eat a piece, even though it was only eight-thirty in the morning. We always opened gifts one at a time, in a circle, starting with the youngest. I always went first, very excited to see what I got. It was fun to give gifts and bring happiness to someone in my family. Opening gifts one at a time taught me to be patient, wait, and enjoy what others shared and received. It was usually noon by the time we had all opened our gifts, and then it was time to clean up the mess and prepare for grandpas, grandmas, uncles, aunts, and the occasional cousin to come. I had fun playing games until dinner was ready.

I loved the way my mom cared for her home, always working to keep it beautiful, and Christmas was the time to show it off. Dinner had to be special and formal, so we had only her best china, candles, crystal, and other items out. The holiday typically included martinis and other cocktails, and as the years went by, dinner was served later and later. By the time it was ready, everyone had tons of appetizers and cocktails. After dinner, we opened more gifts, and the oldest went first. We always had a lot of gifts and a lot of people. Every year my mom would cry when she received a Waterford piece of crystal because they were so expensive and very important to my mom. My dad gave her something special, and some of the children would make handmade gifts or give pictures of themselves or family. We were all entertained by Mom's crying and display of gratitude for the expensive and sentimental gifts.

Mom stated she was abused by her parents and grew up poor. She almost died of diphtheria at the age of twelve. Christian scientists came to pray over her until she could drink grape juice.

According to Kohlberg's Theory of Development, she developed morally divergently from my father. She was also from a different socio-economic class. She made sure she married a man who was financially successful and could provide her with money and the life she wanted. Next, to please my dad, my mom dedicated her attention to the gourmet lifestyle, including the daily cocktail hour. Like a duck on water, my mom had two cocktails almost every evening for as long as I knew her.

A believer in tit for tat, Mom used money as a manipulation power tool, to bargain for what she wanted. *I do something for you; now you must do something for me.* As a parent, she was the Elasta-girl of control— *self-control, mind control, control you, control the house, control everyone with money, control whatever was necessary,* though often in a passive-aggressive way.

As a woman who drank daily, my mom had sudden changes in mood and behavior, making her interactions with me unpredictable. It was difficult for me to be open and trust whether I could receive love from her because I never knew which side would show. Often, she just got louder, and many times humiliated or attacked me with back-handed compliments and rude, cutting remarks. I named it "Perpendicular Love"—*love that showed up in disguise or sideways, from out of nowhere, in unexpected, sarcastic, or passively aggressive ways.* When I was older and told her I was getting married, she said, *"Well, fine hon. I'm sure you'll probably get married at some odd time because normal people get married in June or August. Since you are not normal, you'll marry at some other time."* I often found myself pausing to try to figure out where the thinking came from that would cause a mother to say things like that to her own child.

The cocktail hour was a daily family routine, our time to sit and chat before the prevocational family dinners, which were long and droning. Most took on the characteristics of my dad's personality, moderately to severely stubborn and argumentative. My brother ongoingly engaged him in debates on whatever the topic happened to be. Too many escalated into arguments. Mom intervened to change the subject and stop the argument. Family dinners made for constant entertainment, though they were never fun for me. I was often blindsided by their erratic words and sharp verbal interactions and had to be continually on my toes and protect my heart. Dad typically ended the debate or argument by restating his opinion in a final tone, as if it were fact. Then everyone was quiet for a time and had an alcoholic dessert drink to finish the dinner. Later, no one remembered the arguments or what was said. I assumed this was the way all families spent dinner, but I felt I had to keep this secret from my friends.

For whatever reason, my parents were narcissistic. They communicated through control, demands, rules, and ego-based logic. The punishment never fits the crime, always too cruel for the action or mistake. While hiding behind a door, I saw my brother get the whip for getting an F on his report card. Constantly compared with my siblings, my mom would tell me things like, *"Your sister got straight A's; Your sister got an A in algebra."* I felt I was continually subject to a comparison of one kind or another, rarely validated for my thoughts, actions, talents, or efforts. They were rarely complimentary. I was routinely told that I knew nothing, either from a sibling or parent. I was increasingly riddled with uninvited expectations, comparisons with my siblings, and standards from my mom that I must meet at all costs. With her continual demeaning innuendos and criticism and my father's abrupt bullish teasing and tyranny, I became afraid of my parents. Never knowing what surprise was coming, from which direction, and from whom, but knowing it would come, I worried about it coming and waited for their jabs daily.

My siblings had the same effect on me, with their manipulation, betrayal, deceit, mocking laughter, and one-upmanship. My brother would tell me that I was gullible or laugh at me. I was the only one who was not allowed to do what everyone else did. I was *"not old enough"* or *"not good enough"* or *" too young to know anything,"* or *"not smart enough."* They set the barometer: perfection. I felt I could never measure up.

Despite it all, as a youngest child within the family, I had no other choice. Conform and adapt, or be crushed. So, I learned to cope by brushing it all off as *just them being them*. In the process, however, I developed a habit of screening myself. As a manipulated, controlled and suppressed child, whose thoughts, needs, feelings, and desires did not matter, I stopped expressing my true self at a fairly young age. My energy flow slowly closed, and the conditioning induced coping mechanisms that had taken hold began spouting beneath the surface. Other than **writing on my pillow,** I had no outlet to channel my feelings of fear, anger, sadness, and unworthiness, and I retaliated against my best friend on occasion.

While I suffered as the scapegoat, another part of me was afraid for my mom, afraid that one of my siblings would hurt her. My siblings had been trained well by our parents, and as they grew older, they grew stronger in their offensive abilities. My sister could eventually overpower my mom in her manipulative energy, words, and actions. There were periods when I knew my mom was hurt. I felt afraid for her but powerless to help her. As a child, I thought that she should be able to handle herself. She was an adult. But this evolution was the result of her and my dad's own creation and the byproduct of the narcissistic, abusive, alcoholic home.

Alcohol played a major role in my development when I was about twelve or thirteen wanting to participate in the nightly cocktails. On one of these celebratory weekend evenings, I brought our birds out of their cages. They flew to the martini glasses and started dipping. An hour later, they were doing flips inside their cages, and everyone was laughing. Our dog lapped up some beer and walked sideways for a while. The more cocktails my parents had, the more their behavior changed. My dad would make faces, forcing his eyes and mouth open. By midnight or one am, my mom would be walking around wearing her see-through negligée. Some of these nights were good and fun. Others were just embarrassing for me. They were functioning, so there was not anything for me to do. Just endure.

Having only my experience to draw from, I assumed that my life was pretty normal, though I felt like I never fit in anywhere. Not at home, not in other groups, not in my friends' families. The mother of one of my friends was the den mother for our Bluebird troop, so the meetings were at her house. I enjoyed going to their home. After spending time there and at other friends' homes, I began noticing how different their families were, how differently they lived. They didn't have all-day drinking beach days and champagne brunches, followed by cocktails on the weekends as my family did. They went to church. At a point, I stopped wanting to bring my friends over.

I worried about my parents' drinking. When I was younger, hearing the icebox opening was my signal that dinner would be within an hour or two. As I got older, and my siblings were either out or had moved out of the house, the icebox opened three or three and a half hours before dinner. Some nights I heard it much earlier, like two-thirty in the afternoon. I often felt ashamed and guilty that both parents drank too much. I thought that most people do not have multiple drinks every night of the week.

CHAPTER 2

A Product of Habit

In high school, I failed to make the color guard squad, an expectation fairly high on my mom's list. Fortunately, one of the teachers recommended that I try out for varsity cheerleading. There were only four female positions, and hundreds were trying out. Four thousand students voted. I made the cut. As a gift, my parents gave me a lovely necklace with a miniature megaphone. I loved it and wore it every day.

Though I had been encouraged to develop the drinking habit with my family a few years earlier, on my sixteenth birthday celebration, my mother made an announcement, which made it official. My very first boyfriend, a wrestler, was there to celebrate it with me. He was the best-looking fellow I had ever seen, strong and so sure of himself. I was attracted to that. We'd drive around partying in his friend's van with the hippie carpeting on the side-walls and sixties beads dividing the front seats from the back. He introduced me to marijuana. I used the megaphone on my neck-lace as a roach clip. We went to parties that offered different types of weed. I never knew what kind it was or where it was from, which made me nervous, but he assured me that it was Hawaiian and good stuff. I had tried different types before with him, so I trusted him. One Saturday, we smoked some that had been laced with something else. I was not into hallucinogens, and it made me feel very uncomfortable, out of control. Paranoid, I began seeing forty TVs. That and subsequent experiences recommitted me to the tried and true cocktail.

My mom and I argued when we had too many cocktails. She just did not make sense. But she was my mother. I had to obey her. That seemed so unfair. I tried to get back by being manipulative and cunning and attacking her back. It was my self-test to hold my own and see how much I could get away with when she was too drunk to notice. I hated myself for being so nasty, but I was caught up in the dysfunctional dynamic and couldn't seem to stop.

I was given private driving lessons to prepare for the DMV test. My mom asked my older brother to help me practice the three-point turns in a parking lot. She had raised me to trust him, but I felt very nervous. He was serious, impatient, and judgmental, definitely not patient or supportive, and quite prone to chronic teasing. My mom told me that everyone passes their driver's exam with a hundred percent and made a big deal out of me getting a decent score, a.k.a. a hundred percent. She gave me five pre-exams and instructed me to study both the questions and answers, so I would get a perfect score. I developed a neurosis over not missing any questions. I took the test and got one answer wrong. I had glasses of my favorite, Soave Bolla, that night to quiet the critical self-judgment. I think that was about the time I started picking and cutting myself.

My childhood blessing was to be born after my siblings. Being the youngest, I spent the most one-on-one time with my mother as my siblings moved out one by one. Sometimes she talked about changing my thinking, a mindset she had learned from her father. Both parents grew slightly softer in ways, and I did not suffer the same severity and strictness my siblings and I had endured earlier in my childhood. After they had all moved out, the nightly dinner arguments stopped. But my dad was still a rude prankster. After a few cocktails one night, he pulled a chair out for me to sit down for dinner. As I started to sit, he pulled the chair out from under me, and I fell on the floor. He let out a big laugh.

My mom became even more focused on being a gourmet cook

and making certain that each meal was perfect. She started buying extravagant and uniquely exotic kitchen tools and treating Dad and me to some of her best, most exquisite dishes. She took a great deal of time to put dinner out, and the cocktail hour grew into three. As dinner was served later and later, she told us that we were now eating later "European style." The longer dinner took to be served, the faster I got at drinking.

Tom Collins was my first date drink outside my family home, when I was barely seventeen and on a date with my next older college boyfriend. After that, I could not be anywhere without my friend, King Alcohol. I became an active drinker, drinking at college fraternities and out of kegs with my friends—a big deal and great fun. I even took my Bacardi bottle with me when I went to the hospital to have my tonsils removed.

The energy around money changed around that time as my dad's career took a slippery step. Over many decades of hard work and strategy, my dad had built his father's business and its profits—in anticipation of owning the company when his father retired. He developed operations, marketing, planning, and budgeting, hired a general manager and vice president of sales, and developed the sales force—both in the United States and internationally—with two locations, many salespeople, and many agents who carried his line.

One day, it was revealed to my dad that his father planned to sell the business out from under him. My dad was forced to hire an attorney to protect his position and his future. I didn't understand how a man could do that to his own child and thought my grandfather was awfully greedy to sell the company that my dad had designed, built, and automated. My dad was exquisitely stoic, but it was hard for me to watch. In the end, his attorney negotiated a settlement and the position of CEO for my dad, along with a very handsome salary, pension, retirement, insurance, benefits to exclusive clubs, and a new company car every two years. I got my parents' old car. Finally, something just for me.

As CEO, my dad continued to make very important business relationships around the world, including a famous Italian shoemaker who invited me to select a new pair three or four times a year. Another perk of his position was free and unlimited supplies of alcohol. He brought cases of all kinds of booze home, including Bacardi, wine, vermouth, vodka, and others. As a thank you to my dad for helping save his business, one of his friends put $800,000 in a Swiss bank account for my dad. In a beautiful gift to us, Dad set aside equal shares for my siblings and me. We had some wonderful creature comforts during those years (I sported some very nice clothes from the nicer department stores like Bullocks Wilshire, I. Magnin, and Bonwit Teller and took a modeling class at Bullocks). Ironically, although his attorney was able to negotiate all of that for my dad, had my dad's father passed the company down to my dad, he would have been filthy rich.

With the courage from the victory of making varsity cheerleader under my belt, I ran for and won the position of student body corresponding secretary. I also made the principal's honor roll and high school sorority. High school became the most enjoyable time for me. Becoming a leader not only provided an avenue for me to serve the community, but it also provided recognition, which supported my self-esteem, and I began to feel better around my peers.

The insidiousness of the disease of alcoholism was such that, for a time, I was able to balance daily drinking and partying on the weekends with maintaining my school academics and leadership. Noticing other friends partying justified my drinking and made me think I was okay. Simultaneously, fears of becoming a troubled, fearful person brewed beneath the surface. It became increasingly more difficult for me to balance my emotions, my ego, my reputation, and the two separate worlds I was living in.

Alcohol brought me an instant sense of ease and comfort that allowed me to escape from my worries and calm down. My feelings of restlessness, irritability, orneriness, neurosis, and malcontent subsided, and I could face myself and life. Little by little, items I previously valued became less important, and the partying became the bigger goal. Using the beautiful megaphone necklace my parents had given me as a roach clip was a symptom of my shifting values.

The internal juxtaposition between partying with a depressant and being a fun girl who loved to party became especially painful one Friday night. Caught drinking in our cars at Jack in the Box, we were told by the police to go home. We pretended to leave and snuck around the corner, thinking no one would see us. Twenty minutes later, the police pulled up, got out of the car, pulled my left arm hard, and spun me around, then handcuffed me and shoved me headfirst into the back seat of the patrol car. They told the other kids to go home and drove away with me. I started crying, knowing my parents would kill me if I went to jail, but I was more horrified because of the strictness and fear I was raised in. The officer who was driving turned around to look at me, asked me some questions, and asked for my address. They took me home, dropped me off, and left. I was stunned. Luckily, the house was quiet, so I went straight to my room. I knew that my reputation as a school leader would be seriously tarnished. The intense embarrassment was threatening enough for me to have a talk with myself and regain self-control, though temporarily.

For my high school graduation, my parents gifted me a trip to Europe with the Foreign Study League. I could earn three college units in the summer before college. I was excited, but I didn't want to go alone, so I asked a friend who loved to party, though she did not have the same fixation and compulsion that I did. She was a year behind me, and she had two brothers who were alcohol and drug addicts. A large group of kids from another school went with us, but she and I roomed together. We bought a carton of cigarettes in Rome because that was the cool thing to do. We visited a variety of pubs, smoked many cigarettes, partied a lot, and had a ton of fun. I learned the history, cultures, and customs of five different countries and visited numerous well-known sites.

I was surprised how rampant the underground drug scene was in Amsterdam. I felt safe and in control of alcohol. It was a legal controlled substance, and I was raised with daily drinking, so I didn't see anything wrong with drinking. My friend, on the other hand, wanted to buy some weed. That was a world I had previously explored and did not enjoy. Our teacher told us officials would be checking for drugs and made sure we left clean, but we were never checked.

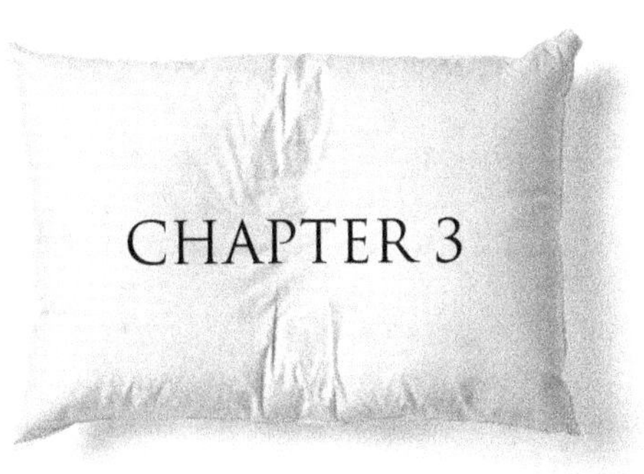

CHAPTER 3

The Invisible Line

After graduation from high school and attending a local college I moved to Isla Vista to attend the University of California at Santa Barbara. Joining the second sorority encouraged frequent partying activities and drinking fun, and I became more focused on daily drinking. I went to bars with various friends for disco night on Mondays and Tuesdays where wine liters were half price. I could not find friends to go out with me both nights until I met Andrea.

Self-managing was both a science and an art. I had another boyfriend who loved marijuana, so I started using it just to balance the effect of the alcohol, so I could handle more. I went to great lengths to become a chemist, reaching new heights in my ability to tolerate higher amounts of alcohol. *Part of the recovery book in chapter three discusses how one tries to control and enjoy drinking with these and other tactics.*

Back at home, I went to a party that started at 11:30 in the day. After finishing the keg, I left the party at 5:30. I made a left turn, and the car wheels folded, so I decided to pull over and rest. I woke abruptly to a scary knock on my window and a police officer asking, *"Are you ok?"* I must have smelled to high heaven. They asked if I had anything to drink. I told him that I had one or two beers. The officers drove me home, red lights on and whirling bright enough to light up the whole street, shining right into the house windows where my dog was sitting and barking. As usual, the lady across the street was spying. She knew everything that was going on when we were outside. The look on my youngest older sister's face—the look of the codependent—asked, *"So, what have you done now?"* Most people have a sibling who might keep a secret. Not mine. Any chance to make me look poorly and she was on it. The next day, I took my car to the gas station for Jess to fix it. Jess was the owner of a well known corner gas station back in the seventies who pumped my gas, cleaned all my windows, checked the air in my tires and checked the oil in my car and fixed anything I needed.

I gave him my Dads credit card. He repeatedly greeted me with, "Hi ornary!"

In my second year of university college, I roomed in an off-campus dorm. Before going out for the evening, I had three to five "getting dressed drinks," so no one would know how much I consumed. I wrote a paper on the subject of alcoholism for a sociology class. I wanted to find out about it without anyone knowing. I thought no one would suspect me. I discovered that it was the third most prevalent disease after cancer and heart disease. When my outspoken New York roommate said, *"You are an alcoholic,"* I responded, *"Not me—you must be talking about my dad. He is an alcoholic. Not me."* I figured she did not know what she was talking about, because she was just as bad—*if not worse*—using hallucinogenic mushrooms every weekend.

Since third grade, I had come to believe that I was not fast or good at comprehension, and test-taking created even more anxiety. I believed that my inability was a symptom of low intelligence, having no idea that it was an actual skill. Instead of seeing things for what they were—tasks—I personalized everything. Increasingly stressed and overwhelmed, I feared I would not be able to complete what was in front of me. I didn't know how I could read all those pages. I read the data two and three times, to make sure I could understand it. Taking all those units and drinking nightly became challenging. Sitting in classes was like sitting in an auditorium, hoping I'd understand what the teacher was saying up on stage and then getting on my bike to travel to the next class in another auditorium, but with twenty thousand bikes. I was riding each time with Bacardi in my backpack because I could not be without some drink, pill, or fix to feel secure.

My roommate wrote a letter to me, explaining why I should be displaced from the dorm. As I read it, I was brought back to my childhood. The letter typified what I grew up hearing from my younger older sister, with almost the exact words, handwriting, and reasoning. I recognized the painful similarity in my attracting a person nearly identical to my sister, in an eerily familiar situation, sharing a room in a bigger "house," and having no choice to go elsewhere. My mind and body were too steeped in chemicals to identify the nature of this circumstance and the source of my discomfort, but I saved the letter.

I looked up to and loved my oldest sister and her husband, and when they decided to move up to Santa Barbara and offered temporary use of one of their bedrooms to me, I gratefully accepted. I had been in an uncomfortable dorm situation, and after staying with them, I felt much better. I felt at home.

Immediately, I settled into the habit of daily Bacardi during school breaks and the nightly cocktail hour, smoking cigarettes offered by my sister and her husband. My parents had taught me that nightly cocktails were associated with elegance, success, and conviviality, though I could only afford the cheap Almaden. After a few weeks, I became a little paranoid that someone would notice me going to the same liquor store around the corner from Francisco Torres dorm every day or two and buying a gallon of Almaden.

The first year passed, spending a few days a week at my sister's drinking cocktails at noon alone. After a few drinks on one warm sunshiny day, I had a strange feeling inside, and I thought to myself, *Am I an alcoholic? Maybe I should call a twelve-step program.* The thought quickly changed to, *No, I'm not that bad. It's just who I am.* I drove back to the Francisco Torres dorm on that warm sunshiny day, past the local liquor store, turned left into the parking lot, and ran into a parked car. A half a dozen people standing in a circle looked right at me. I needed to cover up my mistake quickly— *a reoccurring theme growing up*—so I got out of my car, wrote a note, and put it on the windshield of the tan Ford, making sure the people saw me. The note said, *"Sorry I hit your car."* That's it. I did not leave my name or number. I got back in my car and drove to another area of the parking lot, out of view of the people, drank another Bacardi and coke, and went to class at three o'clock.

I thought the world of my oldest sister's husband. When I was eleven, and he was drafted into the war, I had written a poem to him. I prayed, asking God to watch over him in Vietnam. He had always been so jovial and upbeat and was still that way while I was living with them. My sister was always supportive and helpful.

Sometimes, if she worked long hours, she'd make dinner, wash the dishes, watch a TV show, and go to bed. On one of these nights, my sister's husband was watching a soft porn show, and I watched it with him. The next thing I knew, he was making a sexual move on me. Not only did I look up to him, but I also thought he had a great personality and was pretty cute. I thought that perhaps he needed some relief, so I did not want to reject him. I didn't know what else to do, so I allowed it.

It happened only at that time, but I felt horrible. I had betrayed my sister, and I knew it was wrong. I should have stopped him. Guilt and remorse were on me like a tiger, and I could not forgive myself. It became difficult living there and being around her, knowing I was holding this secret. So, I started drinking even more. By mid-sophomore year, my grades were dropping, and I lost time from work because of my drinking. Months later, while drinking in my bedroom, my three-year-old niece walked in to ask what I was doing and if I could come out and play. I felt she had seen me drinking, and that guilt added to my pile.

The next year I got an off-campus dorm with some other women in Isla Vista and a part-time job at Robinsons May department store. Alcohol became my primary motivator in life. My goal was to get my homework out of the way, so I could treat myself to drinks. Most nights I asked one of my roommates or neighbors to go out for a drink. I was so relieved when I finally found a solid friend to go with me regularly and take advantage of the two liters of wine for the price of one. We found men to dance with for hours at a time. We binged on one-night stands every weekend. At this point, I did not care who I slept with. Someone different two or three times a weekend. I slept with more than a hundred men during that time. Later, after I got sober and was working the fourth step in the program, I labeled each of them by number. No way could I remember names.

I started calling in sick with the flu. I'd had too much to drink and could not get out of bed. Soon, work got in the way of my drinking. I got tired of calling in with the flu excuse. So, I quit my job.

That summer, my drinking friend Andrea and I went on a cross country trip. In Cedar Heights, Utah, the fan belt fell off the car, and the fan ate the radiator. We were stuck there for the weekend. I was devastated. In Utah, no one serves or sells alcohol on Sunday. I truly did not know how I was going to survive.

Wine began to taste like water. I had to have alcohol with me at all times, even when I went to Disneyland. Drinking had become my favorite past time, and I preferred to drink alone. I started getting headaches if I didn't have enough to drink. My craving came like clockwork every day at cocktail hour. I had developed a science of combining one half of a joint and a Henry Weinhard beer to maintain functioning at school. Marijuana accomplished two things. It curbed my need for more alcohol, and it prevented a hangover the next day.

I was aware that my parents knew that I had started drinking during the day. When I visited them for a few days, it didn't seem like they drank much. I had to have two or three drinks before joining them for cocktail hour. I tried not to drink during the weekday, because they didn't, and because I didn't want them to know how badly my addiction had a hold on me. But my body had become so dependent that withdrawal filled me with such nausea, tremors, and shaking that I had to leave. How ironic it was—leaving the scene of my perpetrators, out of fear of their judgment. This was my own fear because the voice inside knew I had a problem but not willing to look at it. This was an afternoon in the middle of the week. I went straight to the liquor store for a pint of Bacardi, drove through Naugle's for a diet coke, poured most of the coke out, and filled it up with Bacardi.

Over time, I took fewer and fewer units per semester. I told my parents that I was not going to graduate until June, though I was graduating in March. I wanted them to keep sending the checks, so I could party twenty-four seven. Much of my time was spent at the Idle Hour with my bar drinking companions. I fell into a cycle of drinking too much and feeling so bad the next day that I swore to never do it again. By early evening, I'd feel better, forget how I had been feeling, and begin the drinking. Drinking around the clock, the drink took a drink, never seeing that ever-invincible invisible line I had crossed when my body became physically and uncontrollably addicted. The line is a downhill glide. Once, all perception of reality goes in a downward spiral.

During Christmas vacation, I drove my car down to the Buffum's parking lot in the Long Beach Marina to sit and drink until I drowned nausea, shakes, and neurosis, and I was back to what I determined was normal, and I was able to talk and interact with others. I walked around with bottles in my purse. I put bottles in my drawers. I hid bottles everywhere. I never went without a bottle. I drank the Vodka under the sink at my parents' and refilled it with water. I just wanted to be like my parents. I wanted to fit in. But at more than a quart of Bacardi every day, curtailing that with a half-gallon of Gallo wine almost every night, every night, I had surpassed the alcohol consumption level of anyone my age. Restlessness, irritability, and orneriness had become my norm. *Party on*, I thought.

Most of the time I could not find my car. I got into a lot of one-car accidents. The tree got in the way, and I just didn't see it. I was always on my way to or from a party. I'd just take my car to Jess. He always helped make it look better.

My parents left for Europe for five weeks, and I went straight for their bar, which I saw as *all mine.* Sitting in the sun in their backyard, next to their greenhouse and sunken spa for five weeks was one big party. I played Beat the Clock with a full glass of Bacardi and coke every fifteen minutes. After four or five drinks at a time, I felt like facing the day. I stumbled around, smoking cigarettes I bummed off of others. I drank a case of Bacardi, twelve quarts, in ten days. I finished up their entire bar supply. There were blackouts and periods of time that I could not remember what food I cooked or where it went. I regularly could not remember where I parked my car, walking around the block looking for it. Police drove me home on several occasions. I got into several one-car accidents, bumping into trees, curbs, and other objects. When my parents returned, my dad took one look at my banged-up car and said that it looked like an alcoholic car.

CHAPTER 4

Powerless

One of the most difficult attributes of having a disease is trying to figure out how I got it. The most severe aspect of alcoholism is the denial portion, the aspect of my not being able to see that I had a problem. To date, alcoholism is the only disease that tells the victim he does not have it. The incredible denial inside me was furious. My favorite pastime became my denial that people were noticing. I was in complete denial that I could possibly have a problem. No way. The insurmountable ego was too great to allow me to see myself as I truly was a hopeless and helpless victim of King Alcohol and a child of an alcoholic. All I saw was the party.

As I devolved into a hermit, I became even more fearful of people and places unless I had four or five drinks to take the edge off. Every day I woke up afraid of the future, afraid about where my life was going, not knowing what I was going to do. Life was a very unhappy place for me. I had become neurotic and paranoid. Riddled with one hundred forms of fear—the king of which was the fear of running out of alcohol—I felt trapped in a cage, completely stuck in a downward spiral, with no way out and nowhere to go. I had occasional periods of clear realization of what I had become, but in those moments, the contrast was so staggering to look at that I drank faster, in search of a speedy way into oblivion.

I lost concern for the type of pills I took off the street, which was a benchmark for me. Alcohol was a controlled substance. I grew up with alcohol. It was how I was raised. This was accepted by my parents and my family. Back when I still had a moral internal boundary, drugs off the street in Amsterdam and later in Santa Barbara were a strict no-no. As my frontal lobe became increasingly affected by alcohol, my ability to discern, care, and self-preserve slowly disappeared. By that point, the almighty pursuit of the feeling that drugs and alcohol brought drove me to buy drugs off the street, and I accepted pills and drinks from anyone, not knowing what I was taking.

The building maintenance guy at my apartment complex became my boyfriend. He asked to take pictures of me nude. I said no. But on a fatal night in December of 1979, in the depths of despair in my seesaw realm and riddled with the stink of booze, I crossed the invisible line of my own internal boundary. At 154 pounds of alcoholic bloat with slits for eyes, holding a wine glass naked, I gave in.

Much later, the sister of my high school boyfriend walked by the maintenance guy's apartment and saw my photos plastered all over his walls. Clearly, King Alcohol had taken away the last ounce of my self-preservation. My already low self-esteem hit rock bottom, and the caring of myself had completely disappeared. The self-loathing I had generated all my life from my diseased childhood environment had bloomed, and I literally hated what I had become. At that point, I did not care what happened to Robin.

Not liking what I saw in the mirror, I told myself horrible ideas about me and how disgusting I looked from the years of alcohol, smoking, pills, and thirty-five pounds of bloat, combined with the effects of picking and cutting my skin—not to mention the things I put in my mouth that I called food. I sat, hopelessly and helplessly addicted, in my Isla Vista apartment with drapes closed and Care Unit commercials running, refusing to answer the door. The emotional pain became so great that the bottle became my spirit—my one and only love and my way out of emotional pain. You simply could not hurt me then. I had a backstop.

In the course of a little over a year, I reached the point of being a slobbering drunk, smelling to high heaven, without the energy to walk or get out of bed some days. Most days, I crawled from the couch to the toilet and back, hiding inside the cocoon that was my apartment. I became helplessly chained to alcohol, drinking close to twenty-four hours a day. If I missed a drink for any period of hours, I shivered periodically, sweated, and had the shakes. In a massive depression, I missed many pieces of time. I'd put a nice tender juicy steak in the oven at night and forget that the oven was on. I'd smell burning the next morning, and find a black very crispy ball in the oven, not to mention have a headache and waves of nausea. One afternoon, I walked out of my second-floor apartment and stood on the second-story walkway. It was a very sunny day, but I could not feel any warmth. I looked down at the pool and wanted to jump. Looking at the trajectory, I saw that I could not realistically land in the pool. It looked like I would most likely hit the cement. I asked myself whether it mattered. That might hurt. I thought, *what if I survived?* That would be worse.

At twenty-two, I was a hopelessly addicted, seriously convoluted vessel full of chemicals. Filled with the hideous four horsemen called terror, bewilderment, frustration, and despair, along with thirty-five extra pounds of flabby alcoholic bloat, I was under the weight of the shackles of the locked gate that was my crazed and racing negative mind. I could not remove them, and I could no longer drink enough to get that high that provided the relief I needed. It was at this point, at midnight on the Wednesday of a particularly rough alcoholic episode in February, that my sixty-five-year-old neighbor, Betty, knocked on my door. I was not answering the door for anyone, but when I saw it was Betty, I let her in. She'd heard me fall again and came up to see if I was ok. After dampening a washcloth, she held my hands and sat very close to me on the couch. I could do nothing but look at her, because I was shaking and trembling and dripping with alcoholic sweat. I'd heard her say that she used to help her husband who had a drinking problem. She asked if I would talk to a counselor at Pine Crest Hospital. I said yes. By two am I was in a taxi cab.

CHAPTER 5

Runner Robin

J ohns Hopkins University Hospital developed a set of twenty questions, designed to measure the symptoms of a person to determine whether he or she is an alcoholic or addict. The best time of presenting the questions to the suspected addict is in the morning after a bout. My first impulse would have typically been to bury my skeletons in a dark closet and padlock the door. Sick and tired of being sick and tired, and on that February morning, I was able to read all twenty questions, without running for a drink. Answering truthfully to my innermost self at that magically right time got my attention. I answered "Yes" to seventeen of the twenty questions. I figured this time I passed the test. Yep, sure enough, I qualified. For the first time, I could see my real self and from this true seeing, I rationally and honestly evaluated my innermost self.

I met with an intake alcohol nurse who tried to talk me into checking into the hospital for treatment. I did not want that to appear on my insurance and did not want my parents to find out, so I declined and told her I would detox at home. She agreed and had me watch Father Martin tapes. And detox in my bathroom I did, seeing bugs everywhere. For days on end, I endured a horrible existence.

What I learned, by reading the doctor's opinion on that fateful morning, and over the next few years, is that alcoholism is a three-fold disease. The manifestation of an allergy, it afflicts individuals with a phenomenal craving like no other, and a craving limited to the alcoholic class, never in the average temperate drinker. The *phenomenon of this craving* is stronger than any amount of willpower, <u>*beyond all mental control*</u>. The allergic individuals can never safely use alcohol in *any form* and, once having formed the habit, discover they cannot break it. This results in their loss of self-confidence and reliance upon all things which are human so that their life problems pile up on them and become astonishingly difficult to solve. The alcoholic disease is so elusive that, while the individuals may admit its resulting injuries, after a time, they cannot differentiate real from perceived injuries. They become increasingly *restless, irritable,* and *discontented* unless they can experience the ease and comfort of taking a few drinks. If they succumb, as so many do, they pass through the states of spree, remorse, and a firm resolution not to drink again. This obsessive cycle repeats over and over unless they can experience the third component—*a true spiritual psychic change*, without which there is very little hope of recovery.

Until that day, what prevented me from believing that I was an alcoholic was the picture in my head of a homeless person wearing a brown overcoat and carrying a bottle in a brown paper bag. But there I was, an objective measurement facing me and the seventeen of twenty questions I honestly answered yes to. Much to my surprise, I qualified. I was indeed an alcoholic.

On March 1st of 1980, my mother's birthday, I attended my first twelve-step meeting in downtown Santa Barbara. They told me about a young people's meeting in Long Beach, so shortly after my first meeting, I moved back to Long Beach and began attending my favorite young people meetings held in the Bank of America building in the Belmont Shore area. I was fascinated by the feeling of love and acceptance, laughter, and pure authentic joy. Wow, I was really attracted to these nice people. These very normal, warm, and inviting human beings sent me home with a large big blue book. This was very foreign, but intriguing to me, so I put in on my coffee table.

I had passed the test, but I was pretty sure I was going to fail the program. As I took out my Bacardi that night, I decided to read that big blue book generously given to me. Drinking and reading go nicely together, I thought. Two months later, I called my oldest sister at two am, spouting out idiotic words and making no sense at all. She sent my brother in law to check on me. He came right away and cleaned up his very filthy alcoholic sister-in-law's apartment. I was beyond grateful. The next morning I had the worst hangover in my life. My head felt three feet wide, and I could barely even see.

I did not believe I could stay sober for a night, let alone a whole day. After all, I had become a compulsive, obsessive daily round the clock drinker. Alcohol and substances were my greatest love. I could count on them to take me away from it all, to escape the emotional pain that I had been in all of my life, day in and day out living with my alcoholic family. I was driven by one hundred forms of fear day and night alike. Alcohol was my solution to the soft quietness inside I so desperately longed for, not to mention the only remedy that could shut off my mind and the ongoing "committee." I had long ago become fed up with people who hurt me. I did not ever want to hurt anymore. I was done feeling pain. Alcohol soothed my nerves and calmed me down. Alcohol allowed me to be happy and gave me a feeling of security. Alcohol was the only object I had ever been able to count on to do its job and do it right. As such, alcohol had become my closest friend. Giving up my one and only love would produce extreme heartache, fear, and neurosis. Twenty-four hours would take a miracle that I was certain was absolutely impossible.

On March 27, 1980, I graduated from UC Santa Barbara. My mom wrote on my college graduation picture, *"She finally made it...we got her through."* It never registered in my awareness that others knew. It never registered in my awareness that *I* knew. I thought I was too young to be an alcoholic. The teeter-totter that I was on, blaming everyone else around me for my life, was a precarious one. I used to say that my dad had a problem. I could see that. I could not see myself. I was a childish, emotionally sensitive, grandiose, and somewhat narcissistic human being, with no regard for another human's feelings and circumstance. Even later when I finally was able to see that I had a problem, I admitted it only to my innermost self.

Looking back at my last year of horrible drinking, I wonder how I made it through, not only mentally, but physically intact and having survived. Because I did not know or understand many of life's principles, I spent the first nine months of my recovery just trying not to pick up a drink. From March 1ˢᵗ to October 7ᵗʰ, 1980 I quit drinking six times. Pick up a drink and stop. Thinking I could easily diagnose myself, I decided to limit myself to just one glass of wine and took my rather full glass of wine and sat in front of the TV for a half-hour. It was either the longest half-hour ever, or my glass was way too small. My friend used to say, I could never find the right size glass.

Attempting to make it through twenty-four hours without a drink had me wavering every other minute, blaming them for my problem and then denying I had a problem. Refusing to see me, I thought all of it must be the fault of my parents. Then, seeing me, I could not fathom how I could possibly go without the chemical that relieved me of the thousand voices inside my head. I would blow up. Most of these committee type voices were cantankerous, critical, angry, and negative and, when coupled with the insurmountably gigantic craving, I wanted to find any way out of myself. I wanted to run away from myself. Then, I just wanted to run.

The people in the meetings nicknamed me "Runner Robin." I did not believe it. Alcoholism is the only disease that tells the sufferer they do not have it. I did not think to my innermost self that I truly had a problem. Needing to be completely clean and sober was fine for them, but my life was in control. This was just my way of life. It wasn't my fault. I grew up with alcohol. I was just a partier. I refused to believe that I was an alcoholic.

With twenty-eight days of sobriety, my longest run in eight years, I went to Vegas to see if I could stay sober. At four am, Cuba Libre's were calling so loudly that I had to shut off my screaming brain at four am. Like a kid in a candy store, I didn't have just one. I had maybe six or eight, or more.

Giving up my first and best love (alcohol) of all time was not only hard enough but excruciatingly painful minute by minute. Quitting six times and slipping six times meant detoxing six times. Seeing black crawling bugs up and down my body, face, and everywhere, I could not hide from them. Minute by minute hearing loud sounds and bells magnified both frightened and depressed, terrified and bewildered me. I was confused and dizzy. Even on sober mornings, I could not drive my car, because the hangover was so magnificent, I could not see. So, I took the train.

Each time I quit, as part of the recovery program, I went back to the meeting, stood up, and introduced myself again, as if it was the first time. Months after my first twelve-step recovery program meeting, knowing that I still was not able to stay sober more than fifty-eight days, a sober woman named Nickie took an interest in me and began calling regularly. Very happy, giggly, grateful, and so full of life, Nickie had what I wanted. Her smile and joviality were infectious and quite an attraction, in contrast to my bumbling efforts of self-degradation and disillusionment.

I moved to Huntington Beach to live with my oldest sister for a short time. She took me to listen to Reverend Peggy Bassett at the Church of Religious Science for a few months. Then I moved back to my hometown of Long Beach. Needing a definitive clarification of whether I was indeed an alcoholic, thinking I could diagnose myself, I decided to move back into my parents' home. Trying to stay sober in their drinking environment, I felt pretty strange. The alcoholism was so prevalent and heavy.

On October 7th, a dark and rainy night, I was smoking a joint in the closet of my childhood bedroom of my parents' home, to hide the scent. Sufficiently numbed, I came out of the closet and poured myself a second glass of wine from the small refrigerator I had put in my room, stocked with liquor and other essentials. Sitting at my card table, listening to music, I began melting crayons with the flame from my lighter, making a picture collage to represent my life. Spaced out in my pain-numbing high, I could hear the background sounds of my parents' voices and the icebox opening and closing. The heaviness of the rainstorm was looming and daunting to me, and as I noticed some of the melted crayons on my collage were burnt, I criticized my sloppiness. Outwardly defiant, inwardly, I was a frightened, disillusioned, cynical woman, chained to the grips of alcohol, about to lose my ability to keep going.

It was raining like cats and dogs. Heavy depressing nonstop rain. My parents were nearby in the kitchen talking amongst themselves. I felt separated in the same house. Listening to my rock songs swaying, creating my life picture through melted crayons moving to the music enjoying getting to that right high place. Reaching for my refrigerator in my bedroom to get more wine. Searching for the ability to get higher. I always felt a need to get higher. When I got up and walked over to the refrigerator to pour more wine for myself. From the darkness came an extremely loud, booming, and distinct voice. Though I had never heard it before, without a doubt, I knew it was GOD/Archangel Michael In an indescribably loving distinct and firm voice, He told me that I was having my last drunk. "Really? Just stop right now?" "YES. YOU DON'T HAVE TO FEEL THIS WAY ANYMORE IF YOU DON'T WANT TO." WOW. Instantaneous. Just like that. A dramatic psychic change.

I put on my beige long trench coat and immediately drove to a sparkling recovery lady named Nickie and told her what happened. I was ready. She was unconditionally ready to help me. The next morning, October 8 1980, was the day I began my climb out.

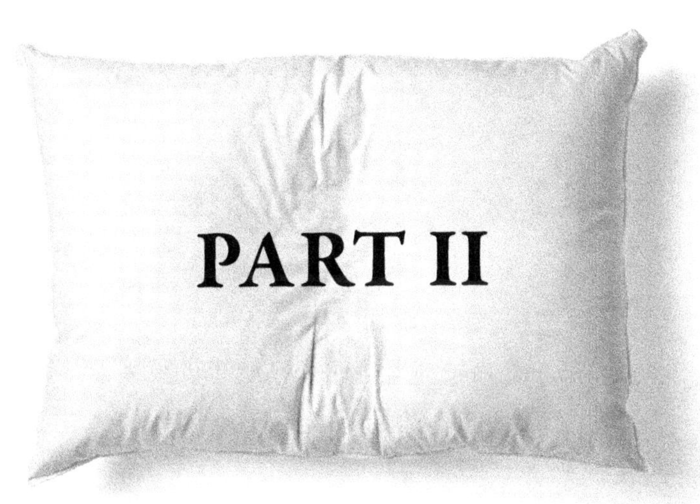
PART II

CHAPTER 6

The Space Between

An angel at my home group recovery meeting named Karen recommended a marriage and family therapist-MFCC, later a Ph.D. who specialized in helping children of alcoholics through her own outpatient therapy program. Smelling to high heaven, a heavyweight slobbering drunk, crawling from the couch to the toilet and back, I had lived drunk 24/7 for three years. I thought, Wow, maybe I have a chance. I scheduled an appointment for the following week, hoping I might make it there.

I was scared to death and very cloudy when I showed up. She had an awesome arrangement, a highly specialized family therapy program for children, before ACA and NACOA existed, with individual sessions, as well as night therapy groups which were a mix of parents of addicts as well as addicts from another family. Her partner was the medical director of a Care unit and a Navy officer psychiatrist.

She had me come early to sit in on the AL-anon, non-addicted codependent, therapy group scheduled before the addicted group. Observing Al-anon, addicted parents, and addicted children in therapy made for interesting group sessions. I watched a nice-looking man keep hitting on the therapist and her repeatedly putting him in his place, by simply using her energy and firm words. I got to see her give boundaries with love, something I had never seen before. It was an amazing process to watch, and I believed that I could trust her. With a very large lump in my throat, I committed to genuine participation.

Then, at my second private session and twelve-step group session, I softly said to the therapist, *"This all seems like brainwashing to me." She responded, "Maybe your brain needs a little washing."* At the ripe old age of twenty-three, addicted and full of alcohol poisoning and not knowing how to recover from a seemingly hopeless state of mind and body, I decided that I would be open-minded and listen to her advice. I then entered into a life and death program to save my life.

Through a profuse amount of reading, meetings, and group sessions, I was advised to become God-Conscious. I was taught about—and questioned—the concept of *becoming the hole in the doughnut. What if I became that? What does that look like?* I was afraid of becoming nothing. That is what my EGO—*Easing God Out*—told me. I was on a new and scary journey. I could not see ahead, had no control, and was unsure of how I might turn out. I immediately went to work and diligently stopped the twelve-inch curls—*aka alcohol*—one minute at a time, one day at a time, in the present moment.

All the while, I wondered how I would keep worried away from my thoughts. I had push-pull, yes-no stay sober conversations in my head twenty-four/seven. Coming from a dysfunctional ego-centric upbringing, I did not know how I could change my insides. Repeatedly, I affirmed, *"Presently, minute to minute, God works through me for his good, every waking moment. Make me a channel of thy peace."* As I did, I felt God (Good Orderly Direction) working through me. With one individual therapy and one group therapy each week, along with regular twelve-step meetings, I progressed from barely making it through the daylight to putting days and nights together with no alcohol, pill, or fix.

Although the process was amazing, it was far from simple, or brief, or permanent. I had brought to the table everything that was me, including an inferiority complex, a lack of self-esteem, doubt and uncertainty about myself, and deeply embedded feelings of not measuring up to standards, ingrained in me by the conditional beliefs I elected to be raised with. I had lived drunk for several years and under the influence of alcohol since I was twelve. Having also become somewhat narcissistic, I had no regard for another person's feelings and position. With absolutely no life tools, I had no concept of reality. Receiving the transmission of my parents numerous fears.ie, growing up during the depression, etc. I was vehemently frightened. I had grown up frightened. I remained childish and emotionally sensitive until I got sober. I felt the feeling of being alone with feeling extreme and chronic ingrained shame of what I had become. During my first few sober months, when someone used a strong tone with me, I cried. Mostly afraid of what I might become. I was afraid to look at my own desire's goals and needs.

If I wanted to stay sober and stay alive, I had to make a commitment to being sober for twenty-four hours and to be open and willing to do what was asked of me. I followed the specific program requests to a T—mostly out of fear and a desire to change—knowing that every waking moment without sobriety was a belly full of booze and a crazed mind. I had to learn the meanings of things all over again. I had to learn a lot more than I could imagine. Cessation of drinking or using drugs was but the first step away from a highly strained, abnormal condition. A few things seemed to help, following that blue recovery book—*my bible.* Visiting with others in the same condition, day in and day out, I learned about faith, "trust in God", "clean house", and "work with others". In between learning methodic breathing, someone taught me seemed to help.

I'd always been a hyper child, busy and running around. For the majority of my life, I felt as though I were on internal over-drive. During the early stages of my recovery, I could not sit still, with excess energy scattered throughout my mind and body, like when you just have the wiggles and don't know what to do about it. Replacing alcohol with coffee didn't help. It was impossible to sit still enough to meditate. So, I started to run around the block.

Alcoholics are enthusiasts. I became an enthusiast and began running around the block of my parents' home. I never considered myself an addicted smoker of sorts. I could take it or leave it at most any given time, but it seemed to calm my nervousness. So, I bummed a cigarette off of the people at the recovery circles. After I learned to run without getting winded, I ventured farther than a block. Getting out and running had the effect of loosening all my neurosis and releasing the neurosis from my skin.

Yet, I wasn't applying any of my outer actions to my insides... until those minutes when my head took off into fear, and I went back and forth with all kinds of imaginings. When I did return to faith, it quickly shifted to fear of the unknown, walking around in a film of wondering, Am I going to make it through today sober? What is in the Spiritual Toolkit that I can use to stay sober through the 'what ifs?' My insides rattled. I still picked at my skin, especially on my face. Reverting back to one minute at a time, I'd do only what was in front of me. Looking beyond was overwhelming. I was told by an old-timer (a long-time sober woman) to chant, *"Of myself I am nothing, God could and would if he were sought (doeth the works)."* That felt ok, not too religious. I had stepped away from all that religion. From my earlier perspective, *there could be no God If I was in this position.* My spirit had been in a bottle. Now my spirit was gone. I was bare. I felt stripped. I walked and moved on true blind faith, not knowing what tomorrow might bring.

Trying to just feel ok with not filling up the space that was newly empty, open and raw, I thought the worst, by default. Was I going to become the hole in the doughnut? What will become of me? Critical thinking and judgment were my upbringings. With no buffers for the first time, trying to find my first job, I was scared out of my mind. My hairs stood on end. My nerve endings were firing on all cylinders. It was a second by the second challenge. When I did land a job, I couldn't do it well or hold it long. Mostly afraid of what I might become, I was afraid to look at my own desires' goals and needs. Because I did not know who I was.

Many days and nights I looked for differences rather than similarities. I was told to look for the similiaities not the differences. I was bewildered sober for a while. Regardless of the depth of soul searching, one can only search and receive if the pathway is clear. Trying to see and understand the infinite with a finite mind is challenging. My humanness often stopped me from hearing or seeing the truth and sometimes still does today. I often did not know how to get out of my own way. I knew nothing of speaking directly to God. I prayed without knowing. I had faith but did not know which way to turn. My vision was to stay sober through each twenty-four hours to make it to the next meeting. Days and nights. Even in the background of my mind with the somewhat loud obsession calling me. Sobriety is first, everything else, second.

At eighty-two days sober, there must be a higher force because I had quit drinking one day at a time. During the break at a Twelve Step convention I attended with my sponsor, I ran around the block. Attendees were standing in large groups smoking. Happiness abounded. Yet, I did not feel that. Space was open inside me that had previously served as a container to hide my self-hatred. Out of a desire to fill that space, and to help me stay sober living in my parents' alcoholic home, I entered into my first sober relationship. I met him while sitting in a jacuzzi one night after a convention. He was sixteen years my senior He asked me to go away to visit a friend in Jamul, California. I felt like a teenager again. My new sober girlfriend cautioned me that the relationship will change, that we will no longer be friends. I didn't know what she meant.

At Christmas time, my first impulse was for no one to find out, to literally bury the skeletons in a dark closet and padlock the door. Instead, I opened the door and walked into my fear. My family is drinking and behaving crazily. Vibrating and shivering, I'm riddled with oppressive fear throughout my mind and body, and feeling more disturbed as the night went on, with no substance to soothe my nerves. My boyfriend was slightly crude, which was embarrassing, but having him by my side was my rock. I knew, absolutely and without a doubt, that I would have instantly picked up another drink had he not been by my side. My parents and most of my family had five, six, seven, eight martinis and then dessert cocktails. Carrying on with the tradition I had lived through from the age of four, each person opened one present at a time. Reliving the emotional stabbing barbs masked as "teasing" was extraordinarily difficult as an already sensitive person, but especially so as a newly sober alcoholic with no substance to buffer me. With dinner still four hours away—at nine o'clock, if we're lucky—glasses are clinking, and ice cubes are rattling. People are getting up and down continually to refill at the bar, acting as though they care about each other, but don't. Often funny, humiliating, shameful, and tragic, that Christmas was no different from the previous twenty years, except for me. I was the sore thumb. No one else had changed. All of my sober neurosis fired from deep inside to the surface of my crawling skin, fully exposed. Overwhelmed by an obsession for relief from anywhere comes over me, much greater than anything I have ever experienced. Others have talked about pacing the floor. I knew I was emotionally unsafe at that very minute. Exposed, raw, and tender, I was a mouse in a lion den, waiting to be devoured.

From my stone-cold sober eyes, I could feel and see the extreme neurosis. Perhaps the years of living with me as an alcoholic was making the co-dependents abnormally neurotic. The alcoholic's past becomes the main asset of the family and, frequently, almost the only one. Perhaps the alcohol was my family's longing for security and happiness. That view is self-centered and in direct conflict with the new way of living sober. My mom had been a duck on the water every day of her life and put a blanket of outer calm on top of it. My family was possessed by the idea that future happiness can be based solely on the forgetfulness of the past. Cover Robin up. Cover everything up. Just cover it up. We are an imagined family -- in many ways, we were the family my mother had imagined.

I was told that, no matter how little sobriety time I had, talking with another female who was at the beginning of recovery, would help both of us. By helping another with less sobriety, I could have a chance to stay sober, whether she did or not. This is the win-win model of success. I was also cautioned not to measure my insides to others outsides. I had measured how well you looked on the outside by how I felt on the inside, but by this comparison and my low self-value, my appearance never felt good enough, no matter how it looked to others. In asking another sober person for a reality check on my thinking, I learned that we cannot see another's insides unless they share their feelings and so my method of measuring was self-defeating.

As I took it one day at a time, my constant mantra remained, *"I only have twenty-four hours."* A younger man helped me to set a goal of staying sober ninety days and nights in a row. In time, I reached the point where I was able to follow the requirements and requests for my sobriety. Doing this at age twenty-three brought me to the point of having had to work through those moments that were long and painful. When I got to the other side, not only did I feel much better for the accomplishment, but I also was in a position, for the first time in my life, to help others to stop drinking, using drugs, and staying stuck. When you stand up at the podium and bring light to others by sharing your transformation, what also changes is your vibration. This is very attractive to the user, abuser, and depressed person because it is the vibrational change that they are able to see and feel through their foggy eyes and mind.

In addition to changing my habits, health, and perception, I felt compelled to satisfy the curiosity of my mind. At every corner, I learned that changing my thinking was the key to my new life. I wanted to open my ability to learn a different way of life, to find out what was possible. In every twenty-four hours, I fed my mind with workshops and teachings of thought leaders like Denis Waitley. I attended Zig Ziegler seminars and Tommy Hopkins sales success workshops.

I listened weekly to Reverend Peggy Bassett. I participated in EST and Millionaire Mind seminars.

1980 was the beginning of my rebirth, in more ways than one. At the beginning of my sobriety, riddled with shame and degradation being depleted of all confidence and self-esteem, because I had hated what I became. By following what I was told—*keep the faith, trust in God, clean house, and work with others*—within the first six months, I learned the spiritual principles which still speak to me today, and how to stay in them. I learned that I could plan or set a goal, but as soon as I pictured being that movie star or looking to be a famous something or so and so, my ego was in the way and I was no longer on divine purpose. If I was operating as that hole in the donut, I was developing and becoming a quality vehicle for my higher power to move through. I had committed to being God-Conscious while staying sober one day at a time. That meant being aware, awake, and deliberate.

CHAPTER 7

Father Time

At the end of my eighth month of sobriety, I was clean and clear enough to notice the ice cubes rattling when my dad opened the freezer at five-thirty am and the intermittent trembling of his hands. I'd ask if he was ok. Of course, he'd say he was. In therapy, I had shared my experiences of how every time someone had suggested that I was an alcoholic, I always responded that they must be talking about my dad. I knew he was an alcoholic. Through my sobriety and spiritual development, it became alarmingly clear to me that I felt I had to help him. My buried childhood dreams of a different life for him were resurfacing. One day, after sharing my concern, the therapist took me seriously and offered to do something about it. My secret dream could actually happen? At that moment, I didn't believe it, *"Yeah right. dad will never go to the hospital."* She said, *"Not unless we ask."*

I knew I'd have to pay for the intervention if I wanted it to happen. So, I set up a payment plan with my therapist truly a professional interventionist and went to work every day with a glimmer of hope. Not long after that, my therapist scheduled an appointment for all family members to meet and participate in the intervention. I could not worry about what people thought. I knew my dad needed help. We did a surprise intervention on both my parents. My mom said no. My dad said yes.

As CEO, he informed his trusted one executive that he would be taking a month's leave, in order to go into the hospital. In the last week of July 1981, he admitted himself into a thirty-day in-patient treatment at Care Manor Hospital of Orange. His room-mate was an NFL Football player, and my dad was a football fan, so that worked out well. He was bussed to Twelve Step meetings at Hoag Hospital. He befriended a man named Jim, and they sat together every Saturday night. A journey where the heart listens and the heart speaks.

After he completed his hospital stay, we went to dinner and a meeting each Saturday at first. My mom explained that she did not mind because it gave her a chance to be alone. She was fantastic at working on her own healing and worked with her own mental thoughts day in and day out.

A believer in Christ and raised by her parents (who historically were very mean to her) but were a form of Christian Science and Grandpa, later on, was a member of the Fullerton Religious Science church. Mom later invested her time on Sunday mornings going to Unity Church or the Church of Spiritual Living.

I had precious times with my dad at those recovery meetings. Not only did I not take a drink, but I also did not desire to take a pill or a fix of any kind, prescribed or not, including Vicodin et.al, one exception—when I had dental surgery. I learned early that just a high dose of ibuprofen was the strongest drug needed along with some rest. Bumming a cigarette, the first few years helped me bridge that feeling of wanting to party and the need to stay sober those early sober nights.

CHAPTER 8

The New Runner Robin

Along with my life and death 24 hour commitment to sobriety, I began to run around the block daily. This time, I was not running from myself, but running for myself. Having been conditioned to be a people pleaser, I struggled mentally, with mind busy-ness and voices. Running helped to quiet my mind, forced me to center, focused my thoughts on my cadence, timing, and form, and helped me control my breathing. Running helped me to be able to sit during long meetings and listen calmly. It felt wonderful and centering to run and then sit for a ninety-minute meeting with my recovery fellows and gals. If I ran after work, I could release my frustrations. Daily running helped me be mentally and physically tired enough to quiet the voices and fall asleep at night. Even if I drank coffee or soda at ten o'clock at night, my running ritual allowed me to go to sleep. Most of all, running helped me feel closer to God, a higher power.

So, I started setting a goal. From twelve-minute runs around the block, I increased to a daily half mile. My lungs didn't just ache; they burned. They burned a lot. My throat burned. I was in poor shape. Finally, after months of one-half miles, I felt better. I wanted more of that. I figured if I could do a few steps in my college running class while drinking, I ought to be able to run more, so I raised my goal to a mile. Then two miles. Then three. For three months I ran up to three miles, still occasionally bumming cigarettes off of people.

I eventually ran farther, from Clark to Carson to Bellflower Avenue and then back down to my childhood home in Stratford square between the Long Beach airport and the Los Altos Drive-In theater along with (Go see Cal) I tried a 5K. Someone told me I should run a 10K and suggested I join a running club called The Running Experience. I began meeting people from the running club who would pick me up at 5:45 am to run before work. I ran my first 10K in Seal Beach and received an award for placing in my age group. That was my first experience of real sober fun since I was a child. I felt happy and accomplished. I continued running with the club and set a goal to run a half marathon.

After running the Catalina 18K, I met a very motivating coach and runner who owned the running experience in Belmont shore and put on a marathon training clinic I wondered if I could run that far. I decided to try to run the first Long Beach World Runners Marathon. I ran it in 3:25, the eighth woman to cross the finish line.

I couldn't have a beer with the others after the race, and everyone laughed because I couldn't walk up or down the stairs at work. I didn't care. The feeling of accomplishment was invaluable. I loved the attention, and I loved the endorphins. They hooked me big time. I was a feel-good oriented being, and when I was that invigorated, I felt more vibrant than ever.

That was my first experience being around people who exhibited unconditional joy. No matter what day, no matter what happened, my new happy running friends displayed daily joy.

When the first Seal Beach, California triathlon was announced, I thought it would be a good test for me. I finished as the 5th woman and qualified for the ironman in my second triathlon. I ran my second marathon in Palos Verdes the next year and qualified to run the Boston Marathon the following year. In 1983, with three years of sobriety, I qualified and ran the Boston Marathon.

Running more events with the running club provided a healthy community and some great friends. We traveled to Honolulu and ran the Honolulu marathon, the most fun marathon I had ever run, and the most fun I had had in a long time. The next day, an attractive and super-fast runner I admired asked if I wanted to take a run with him. We ran eight miles.

I ended up tearing my Achilles tendon and went to a wonderful podiatrist in Long Beach, who also was an avid runner. He told me to stay off my feet for eleven days. It was virtually impossible for me to see how I could do that. My sobriety had been locked into my daily running. I became very depressed. It was time for me to adjust my fixed, constrained personality. I became stuck and sad, very sad.

Someone recommended that I swim. I met some fellow recovery people I knew at the pool, which helped me adjust mentally and physically, and I eventually grew to do some master's workouts.

About a year later, I met another marathon runner. He was strong and fast and spoke about biking and how great it was. He helped me buy a very fast bike, and we cycled a lot together. I soon was able to run again. Having looked up to triathletes, I decided to train to enter a race. I went to the gym and worked out on my own until I met a triathlete who became my coach. He was one of the top three professional triathletes of the USTS series then.

He designed a workout plan for me that included logistics and four days of weight training, to start. Sundays were my day off, and

I could eat anything. On Mondays, I ran eighteen miles. Tuesdays, I biked eighty miles Wednesdays, I swam. On Thursdays, I doubled my running workouts and did added weight training.

I set a goal to run one of the races in the Desert Princess World Championship Race, a three-race Biathlon series and won the second race in my age group. My coach asked me if I wanted to train to do really well the following year. I said yes to training for the three-race series. During my training process, to my amazement, I won the San Bernardino short course triathlon as the overall female winner. And I won the whole Desert Princess World Championship series in my ten-year age range group the following year. The value of participating in these three races was that they were staggered. Although I passed up a lot of professional entries, I didn't know where anyone else was in the race, so I was only competing with myself. Thus, my family conditioning of constantly being compared was removed.

On Saturdays, during the long winter days, I ran twenty-three miles and then went to the recovery dances and danced nonstop for four hours. The fantastic part about the first years of my sobriety was the incredible journey with many, many experiences along the way, the setting of the goals, no matter how they turned out, the sheer delight of the crisp bite of cold air on my face, ears, mouth, and eyes on those winter mornings. I trained so many hours each week, met so many new people placed on my path, and formed lifelong connections. I entered over a dozen annual 5 and 10 K's, marathons, biathlons, and triathlons. I beat some of the pro tri-athletes of the time. The wonderful moment by moment aware-ness that occurred during those experiences was unforgettable. Enjoying my journey unfolding, relishing my time with my higher power, and savoring the outdoors, nature, and the earth was a rare kind of energy— a "wow now time," a long way from crawling from the couch to the toilet and back just years earlier.

CHAPTER 9

A Spiritual Experience

I incorporated many changes in the early months and years of my recovery, but none could have happened without the psychic changes—the spiritual experiences that profoundly awakened me.

Whether we're dealing with substance abuse, psychopathic behaviors, manic depression, or other addiction, I am a believer that something more than human power is needed for producing a lasting change and true transformation. Addiction is a physical allergy with a phenomenon of craving and a psychic imbalance and, therefore, not entirely a problem of mental control. All afflicted individuals may have normal intelligence in every respect of the word.

What differentiates alcoholics from others is the phenomenon of the craving manifested with an allergy. My mom always believed this. She had two or three glasses of wine every night throughout her entire life. The phenomenon of the craving is that it overpowers all other interests—children, marriages, careers, fame, anything. The drinking is not to escape, but to overcome a craving that is beyond the ability to be controlled by mental discipline.

Even if abstinence is achieved, without a true psychic change or spiritual awakening, abstinence does not equate with being clean and clear—only letting go of the external fix, be it a drink, pill, or other addiction. Approximately forty percent of recovered alcoholics turn to gamble, sex, food, relationships, porn, or other addiction as a substitute fix. Nine out of ten quit the drink, pill, or fix and are off doing marijuana maintenance or some other mind-altering therapy. One can just stop using, but the self-development remains arrested and often lacks a true and stable moral compass. One must have help derived not only from a human but from a "psychic change" or "spiritual awakening" for a chance at lasting adjustment and success.

After such a change, no promises need to be made, only a decision. A decision to abstain for twenty-four hours with the help of someone, some method, or self-help. Then, we will succeed, and with our success, present ourselves as evidence for the hope of others.

My experience discovering, understanding, and appreciating my gift of seeing spirits became a spiritual experience in my twenties as a result of the recovery principles I earnestly took and diligently embodied.

As I reflect, I count three major events in my life that brought about my spiritual awakening experience, which I define as a sudden or gradual psychic change. My first was the fateful day in February 1980 when my neighbor Betty—known as my "Eskimo," a recovery term for the person who leads you to your first meeting—came knocking on my apartment door at the exact perfect moment of my receptivity, within my alcohol and drug-filled, shame-based mind and body. For most, this experience would have been enough to permanently turn on the light bulb. Not so for me. I was stubborn and hard-headed.

My second significant spiritual experience was on a fateful night eight months later, when a subtle, yet profound and spectacular, surround sound force from out of nowhere spoke to me in a Wizard of Oz voice. This was none less than a revolutionary upheaval, which invoked an instant personality change in me sufficient to generate an earnest desire for recovery. A glimmer of light sparked hope and an immediate call for help.

Because of my previous failures at self-motivated sobriety, my third spiritual experience was a gradual one that began in a moment of my knowing I was an Atheist, but willing to listen. I was willing to go to any length to overcome a disease that literally took me to the ground, and that desire was stronger than my stubborn atheist mind. Slowly, I opened myself to reading the stories about others' beliefs, which resulted in my mindset shifting to align with an agnostic belief. As the hours ticked by with me observing myself not drinking one day to the next, I entertained the thought that there must be something greater assisting me.

I had the sensation of an invisible presence in the room every time I listened to a member talk about willingness. As an addicted and tormented human, I did not yet see the omnipotence of the Divine. With honesty, open-mindedness, and willingness (HOW)—three concepts I had no prior introduction of—I began to see. It took time for me to recognize the Holy Spirit, and with my new eyes, willingness, and recovery steps, I eventually saw that my Higher Power had been with me the whole time. I had to change my behavior, to incorporate a willingness to be honest with myself—a kind of honesty I had never had before with another human being. I had to straighten out all my twisted relationships to my best ability, ask forgiveness—from others and from myself, give of myself to help someone else, and pray. Meditating was not yet of any interest to me, as I could not yet sit still. These changes connected me directly to my inner resource, known as God Consciousness.

One aspect of real faith is a constant awareness of the Divine presence in my various, everyday routines. Another is the awareness that a Higher Power is simply a power greater than myself. If I am to recreate my life, I can start over at any time. If I am miserable, the problem is at the core of my soul and thought process. If there is previous trauma, it must be removed. Ideals must be grounded in a power greater than myself if I am to recreate my life. The lesson is mindfully based transcendence, versus fear-based, immediate, and instant gratification. The goal is non-reactive mindfulness, versus my own certain or uncertain judgment. Success is both total abstinence and a moral and emotional maturity and clarity, as a result of a psychic change or Spiritual Awakening. We look toward success and get there more and more each day. Hence the term, one day at a time. We receive a daily reprieve based on our spiritual condition.

The sunlight of the spirit cannot reach an addicted mind or body. Some say seek peace instead of a fix. I cannot explain how to ride a bike in a way that will guarantee your success at it, but I can tell you that balance is the key. Surrender, for now, your impatience, self-denigration, and perfectionism, and seek satisfaction as often as possible.

CHAPTER 10

Five Years

The first five years of sobriety were sometimes an extremely frustrating, uncomfortable, and faith-testing period. Fraught with extreme emotions, I often fought with my boyfriend, even arguing while driving, swerving and screaming at him to get out of the car. I knew I would have to keep apologizing for my actions. I reminded myself that I had made a decision to stay sober and follow directions. I needed to be humble and willing to learn. My advisor told me, *"When you get tired of apologizing, maybe you will change. Become willing to be willing to change."* Or just pray for the willingness to be willing. That made sense to me.

I asked my Creator to help me learn to be willing. Little by little, the willingness to confide in someone with my secrets became major healing for me. This type of confession is different from a religious confession. It imposes a change of action, to release the habit, and never to be that way again. Here a full release and elimination of my darkness are done through me by my Creator.

Yet, it was not easy, with many steps forward and two steps backward. I walked through serious fears. Even after my dark night of the soul, when my Creator spoke to me and revealed to me that I had a disease of the mind, I wondered, *Am I really an alcoholic? Is this just a phase of bad brakes?* Driving to meetings, I asked myself, *Do I really need this? A lot of my precious time is sitting in these meetings listening to others' experiences. How is this helping me with all of my problems?* I wanted fixes right now—the job, people, supporting myself, dating, staying clean—all spinning inside my head. I spent a lot of time in my mind and taking actions that felt contrary to my conditioned thinking, trying to force myself to think about other things.

There were times I was so negative and uncomfortable that I was unwilling to take action. My early advisor told me that if I didn't want to talk, I should just write—write anything, with no format. *"Black and white does not lie."* I figured I could do that, I felt as long as no one saw what I wrote. This created some space for me to stay sober. After my fifth step, I was advised to take all I wrote at a separate time, and put it into the fireplace. The action was so freeing to my mind, body, and spirit. I was then able to walk as a free woman. I found that if I waited too long to search those dark crevices, take right action, or write that I could become suicidal, homicidal, and/or drink, which would most likely lead to one of three paths: jail, institution, or death.

Fortunately, my recovery group was strict, with reminders to go to meetings three times a week, along with a Sunday gratitude breakfast. For me, a born and bred escapist, the concrete structure of the recovery program aligned with the strictness of my upbringing and secured my inner insecurity and the two decades of inner baggage I carried. I focused only on one day at a time, keeping as busy as I could, including washing coffee cups and emptying ashtrays after meetings. It was a way of life. A good one.

Knowing that I was not alone in my recovery group and that I could call someone for a reality check helped, as did a faith-filled walk with a trusted friend and reading the book *Single and Sober.* It was all about learning to have faith—and changing my environment and routine.

I had to change my friends. I dedicated more time staying with my own people, those who were strongly active and committed. Our group had a lot of fun together, doing plays, dances, and Halloween parties. We visited people in the hospital and went to other jails and institutions to visit and introduce ourselves. We were planting seeds, carrying the message. Having one-on-one time, taking the spiritual strides as directed, I felt close to these people spending so much time together in love, a celebration of sobriety, and laughter.

I struggled to gain employment, as I needed to establish a feeling of confidence in myself that I had never had. I walked around with my long internalized negative tape playing whenever I went to an interview or someplace new where I had to present myself, *You are not good enough. You are not smart enough. You'll never amount to much. You're not attractive enough. You have made a lot of mistakes.* The jobs I landed, I could not do well in or hold for long. Afraid to talk to anyone, I was afraid of the interview, afraid of people, afraid of not knowing who I was or what to become.

A lot of self-help job and career transition experts told me to look at my hobbies. I had put a lot of time, energy, and study into recovery, but I did not know how that could be a hobby. I thought, *What do I look up to?* I had watched those care unit commercials, blasted up high. That gave me a lift many times in my life when I was filled with one hundred forms of fear, not knowing where to turn, locked up in my own cage. All was new to me in this new version of me. I had devoted so much time, money, and energy on my spirit in a bottle and my previous thoughts of me, that I didn't know how to feel comfortable in my new raw skin, in a world of time and space and choices. After many trials and interviews, I found a job. I was grateful and worked by showing up, even though I felt afraid.

People in recovery sometimes called on me to speak without warning, causing anxiety in me. I felt extremely uncomfortable talking in large groups and preferred the smaller groups, so the laughter and shoves, and the old-timers saying hello helped me get through some very long days. One man, Holiday Kent, would run across the street to give me a big hug every morning at six am, as I ran by his house. There was always something to look forward to in the group, and soon I no longer felt alone. I grew to feel a useful member of society and the human race, with something to contribute, for the first time.

I slowly learned to respond, rather than react to the contrast that life brought. I learned how to apply spiritual concepts to my daily life. I did my spiritual readings. I asked my Creator to remove my character deficits. Putting together hours and days helped me to build my confidence. I found and rented my own apartment for the first time.

The feelings of impending disaster that had haunted my daily awakening in the dozen years prior to my sobriety began to dissolve, piece by piece, as I embodied my new lifestyle, free of anger, self-pity, and resentment. As a result of drilling into my newly forming self the need to be willing; to be willing, I laid a strong foundation of willingness to learn, change, and grow. I was taught to change my attitude. AA was altering attitudes. I began to fully emerge myself into attitude-altering resources and experiences, including the transformational EST Weekend and other healings. Through my continual healing process and spiritual experience, I knew that I fully participated in the solution I achieved. Slowly, I learned how to act in a brand-new way.

Being raised and indoctrinated in the Twelve Steps is what made me and some of the others in our small group truly unique. Sober before the age of twenty-five, we were called young people. A common bond and kinship were formed, which helped me gain my newfound family. We saved each other. Recovery taught me *nice* people existed. It was a foreign experience initially, and one that would keep testing and teaching me as I learned to navigate my new life. I saw, felt, and witnessed great events come to pass in my first five years. I cleared the wreckage of my past. I stepped up to help others. And my life changed.

CHAPTER 11

Wash, Rinse, and Repeat

Developed by two men who could not stop drinking, the big blue book of Twelve Steps remains the most successful program, by far, out of all the treatment options for someone who cannot stop drinking or using—*and for good reason.* No matter what life dilemma or relationship challenge I came up against in my first few years of sobriety and beyond and no matter how many times I slipped and had to climb back up, this handbook for life saved my life and continued to do so, guiding me—*unconditionally and without exception*—where I needed to go.

After my fifth year of sobriety, my life quite suddenly and unexpectedly became a shamble. I was single and sober dating. I had been involved in the therapy group alongside many self-help meetings. I felt that I was a good listener and had just accomplished a goal in my job, making thirty in-person cold calls a day to build my photocopier sales customers. I was teaming up with the sales team and writing leases for customers. I was still a member of the running club and ran six miles every morning with a neighbor.

While attending the leadership sales and awards picnic of the 3.5-billion-dollar company l worked for—one of the top ten companies to work for in the US, I met a company manager who took an interest in me. He was going to Hawaii and asked if I wanted to come. I didn't know it at the time, but he was an imposter and convinced the airline ticket agent that he was one of the famous company's board members and to use an alter ID to get us and the others with us on the plane.

I thought this guy was amazing, a magician. So self-confident. After we returned from Hawaii, he invited me to visit him in Florida where he lived. I took two trips out, and he wined and dined me and showed me all the sites on his boat. He offered to be my supervisor in the company if I moved to Florida. I sold my new car, gave notice to my apartment in Belmont Heights, spent close to ten thousand by the time all was said and done and moved. My new boyfriend's mother and female partner shared a home together in Sarasota, where I stayed and paid their rent while they lived on their boat.

Fortunately, I had met a close friend at one of the self-help meetings, because ninety days after Hurricane Elena, I found my new boyfriend and job supervisor with his arm around another girl. Betrayed, sad, and in shock, in a foreign part of the country and knowing no one, I went into culture shock. Having no money and no man, and far from home, I felt like a failure. I was in a place I had never been—intense and constant discomfort and fear, without alcohol to turn to. I felt trapped, stuck. I wanted a drink. Luckily, my new close recovery friend was with me at the exact moment I found out and took me to a dance place called REBOS (spelled backward on purpose). It was a recovery place where they had dances and meetings. She saved my life.

I floundered for a time, feeling hurt. Poor me, *"Poor me, poor me, pour me another drink,"* I used to hear. Self-pity I could not do, but I did not know what to do. I moved to the southern tip of Siesta Key, purported to be the third prettiest beach in the world at the time. I ran on that beautiful beach, swam in the water, rode a bike at the gym, and ran with the running club. I ran races and beat a few fellows, which was something to be proud of. I was from California, and it's much hotter in Florida and harder to run.

A fast runner introduced himself to me at one of the races and chatted with me at another. Late one night, he knocked on the door of my house and came in and raped me. I tried to get away and ran out of my house. As I ran, I realized that I lived at the end of the island. The nearest seven eleven was three miles up the road the other way. It was near midnight, and no one was awake. I'd had met another self-help fellow, but didn't know which house he was in. I didn't know anyone, and the nearest neighbor's house was set way back off the road. So, I went back to my place. There was not much else I could do. He told me that his wife had left him and that he was very angry with her. He took it out on me. I just left my body while he raped me.

I would have much rather used a chemical, be burdened by a gambling habit, or smoked cigarettes than feel the emotional pain of being bullied as I had felt throughout my years growing up. However, I made a commitment to God to not. A beautiful counselor explained that the rape was not my fault.

I went back to work and had to report to the manager who had tricked and betrayed me until a newly hired manager was assigned to me. He was a bigot and a hick and made derogatory comments to put me down, as I was one of the top sales producers. A new girl was making more sales than I because she was illegally modifying the lease termination dates. I wanted to win the sales contest, so I modified one of my lease renewals to get a sale. My new manager was already looking for a way to get rid of me, so when he found out, he turned me in. I had already lost credibility, because I had been in a relationship with my former manager, so I got fired. Through that experience, I discovered that I was a very competitive individual and that integrity was more important than being number one in the company. After much prayer and complaining, filing an EEOC report, nothing came of it.

I told my mom what happened, and my parents flew out two or three times to make sure I was ok during my few years there. I really did not want to stay sober during those devastating experiences. I figured, *If I could stay sober through all of that, I could probably stay sober through anything.*

Sometimes, what appears as a negative reveal a hidden positive that brings great satisfaction. I remembered that there was a service arm of the recovery program that needed help. I found good program people there. I sponsored other recovery people. I spoke when asked to deliver a personal message. I also remembered that I had started a panel meeting for young women at the Metropolitan State Hospital back home in Norwalk, California, so I brought that message to the recovery people in Florida, side by side with other sober women.

If a person I am counting on disappoints me, and I have no alternative place to put faith in, I am doomed to despair. If a person fails me, I can replace that person with another, but humans are fallible. I learned that there must be two things, reliance on a higher power and structure. Relying on a higher power can be known as my creator, Father, or God, Jesus or other. Any personal higher power is acceptable. One of the aspects associated with addiction is loneliness. I have not met a person previously addicted who could succeed in sobriety without some structure. If there is no structure in the addicted person's life, loneliness sets in and the person flounders, eventually reaching for anything, falling for anything or anyone. The structure is desperately needed.

I could have missed it all. I learned great events will come to pass if I stay sober. Caring about how another person is doing is important. Picking up the fifty-pound telephone and making the phone call saves lives. It literally saved my life. The experience of bringing the message of hope and inspiration is a win-win, a two-ended stick that benefits both the giver and the receiver. It is a guide for how to live my life. I was taught to be of service when I first got sober. If I help someone else, I may not find it necessary to use the drink, pill or fix. I remain with an open-heart with courage wisdom and acceptance. Giving is a mindset. Giving and receiving is a spiritual law that I learned at Science of Mind, Ernest Holmes Institute classes. In the process of attempting to stay alive and not use a pill, drink, or fix, I found myself learning Spiritual Devotion.

To stay clean, one must concentrate on sobriety. *To develop any new condition or habit, one must practice. One must be with others who want the same.* I had begun to learn what new habits I must develop and practice daily—*and what old habits I must release:*

Self-forgetfulness, instead of self-pity

Modesty, instead of self-importance

Seeing good, instead of criticizing

Humility, instead of self-justification

Self-valuation, instead of self-loathing

Positive self-description, instead of self-condemnation

Patience and Tolerance, instead of impatience

Love, instead of hate

Forgiveness, instead of resentment

Simplicity, instead of false pride

Trust, instead of jealousy

Generosity, instead of envy

Activity, instead of laziness

Promptness, instead of procrastination

Straightforwardness, instead of insincerity

Positive thinking, instead of negative thinking

Spiritually high-mindedness, instead of vulgarity and immorality

Faith, instead of Fear

CHAPTER 12

Mind-Body-Spirit Life and Work Path

The Lord works through people. After I lost my job in Florida, I sought help from spiritual counselors. They revealed to me that I should be in Medical school. I thought *They're crazy. How could I do that? I don't have the money.* While that was so far from what was in my head, what I knew was that no one else was going to do this for me. I had to take care of the self, mind, body, and spirit. First was my commitment to my Higher Power. The second was my gratefulness for sobriety. A third was reprogramming my thinking and what I thought I could, or couldn't do.

Since I had a sales background, I decided to cold call a recovery company. I walked in at lunch hour. No one was at the front desk. Out walked the Vice President. I told him I wanted to work for the company. He asked me what type of work I did and said they were looking for sales professionals to call on hospital CEO. I told him I could do that. He then told me that the only problem was that the interview was in Newport Beach, California, where their headquarters were. I got very excited and smiled. *I could get back home.* My first interview was by phone, and the company flew me to Newport Beach for my second interview. Of the seventy-two people interviewed, I came in second. They hired a man within. I asked what other work may I possibly do and told them that I wanted to work for them. My thinking was *If the Care Unit commercials had attracted my attention, working to help other addicts and substance abusers would definitely be helpful to my fellow sufferers. I was* interviewed again for a position to help open ten outpatient units for the firm I was hired.

Reporting to the Executive Vice President, I helped open ten freestanding outpatient centers and was responsible for the profit and loss of two of them. I interviewed psychologists at the corporate office. Of the ten, I was responsible for space planning, opening and operating two of the free-standing outpatient units. I became the only Program Director to show a profit in the first year. All other colleagues hired were previous Hospital department heads, which was a requirement for the job. I had no hospital or operations experience, so I felt that I needed to prove myself. I created and developed an insightful marketing strategy within one of their hospitals. I applied what I had learned from volunteering in the unique therapy group I had graduated from. I sat in and assisted at their hospital clinical meetings until they were trained. I requested help from my colleague who was head of the department at the local hospital.

By the time I was twenty-nine—six and a half years after becoming sober—I had become professionally trained with, and one of the top performers at, one of the top ten sales companies in America. I had advanced to the status of the top leaders in the company branch and one of the top ten percent of the sales leaders nationwide. I had become the director and opener of ten freestanding chemical dependency facilities, supervising five professional psychologists, a licensed MFCC therapist, the business manager, and reception. I was responsible for operations, clinical, and business sectors of a large hospital chain, all of which required me to have prior hospital administration and operations experience and a master's degree. I had neither. In a period of one year, I had developed the only profitable free-standing outpatient center coming from the most highly visible company in the well-known 36 billion-dollar industry.

That level of growth and attainment was a peak experience for me, but even more valuable was the fruit of my willingness to serve. From the age of twenty-two upon entering the recovery program, I was trained to be of service to the greater good of the group. Come early; stay late; shake the newcomer's hands; and give my phone number out, in case someone needs help. I learned to put the ego—*aka Easing God Out*—aside. Being of service within the service arm of my recovery program gave me the best chance to save my own life. If I helped someone else, the act brought satisfaction, and I didn't find it necessary to use the drink, pill or fix.

Being of service saved my life, not only as a volunteer in the program but also as an employee of a recovery company and as a program director of two outpatient freestanding facilities. As a result of developing those centers, from space planning to fruition—from a standpoint of being in service—I envisioned, manifested and facilitated the co-creation of a center. Hundreds of people received help on an outpatient basis from each center. Multiply that by centers opened. I saw many miracles unfold right in front of me. I was privileged to be able to witness the eyes of the people graduating from the outpatient centers, to watch the eyes of the women I sponsored foggy and dull coming into the light. From dark to light, I watched the miracles continue for decades. Every individual coming to the light, every act of service, and every miracle count. "The more lives saved and changed for the better, the better our world becomes and the higher the transformation of the planet."

In 1990, God was telling me to do something else. I needed to go back to school. I could not hear my higher power clearly that year and did not have the self-esteem to listen. I did dream and write goals; however, I was striving to survive, making sure I had a job, thinking I needed to keep a roof over my head, be responsible, and all those things we are taught above all the deeper truths. Working for three clinics owned by a doctor and his wife, I brought in so much business from my marketing efforts that a brand-new separate clinic was developed. After accomplishing that feat, I negotiated for more pay. He threw me out and hired a local driver and maintenance man to call on the customers I had generated.

I discovered I had attracted the bullies in the world. But with this discovery, I became aware of how the errors in my thinking had caused that. After years of working to see with new eyes, recover, and heal myself, I learned that I must love and take care of myself. By my tenth anniversary of being sober, clean, clear, and conscious, I had transformed my health and my body. I had changed what went into my body and what I did with my body. I had accomplished tremendous growth and goals, including winning a 10K Recovery race in the overall female category ten years in a row.

I had a knowing that my mission was to help people. A seed had been planted that generated a growing desire in me to help people with their health. I was offered the position of a recovery counselor by my initial therapist. I loved the owners and the counselors of the clinic and dealing with the mindful negativity that the disease brings sounded challenging.

In making these and other self-esteem enhancing strides, I had reached the realization that I wanted more than anything to be an instrument for God, Source, a channel through which I could be of maximum service to God and others. So many occurrences had serendipitously been leading up to direct me on a new path.

Waiting at the traffic light in my hot blue Camaro to get on the 405 freeway at Studebaker road and a large company truck approaching behind me was not slowing down. I watched in the rearview as he hit his brakes too late. About to be smashed, I gripped the wheel and turned to look, bracing myself for the impact. The doctor of chiropractic told me that was the worst thing ever—turning and bracing. He also told me something I was not expecting. Based on the speed the truck was going and the impact, I should not have a fractured vertebra. Something else was wrong. After a slew of tests; X-rays, blood draws, nerve conduction tests, he informed me that I had chronic fatigue syndrome. This was no typical chiropractor. He had an MD from France and a Ph.D. in Nutrition. He was a special one, warm, gentle and made everyone feel special. I was impressed. Something in me lit up, and my self-healing began.

I did not know it until I knew it, but I was being guided to step fully into the field of energetic medicine and healing. Helping the whole person, Body Mind and Spirit, seemed a divine way of being in service for the health and wellbeing of my fellow man. I decided to train to be an acupuncture and oriental medicine physician.

In part of my academic years, I helped my mentor in the acupuncture clinic. In 1992, I was healed by my mentor of a few issues and realized what an incredible medicine this was. In 1992, as an intern, I began taking care of my parents with Oriental Medicine. Initially, I encountered miracles with my father and mother which became great events. One of the first was my father even considering this unusual alternative medicine to help and to even consider it to help him in the 1990s. But Dad had gone to many MDs and he explained no one could help resolve his intermittent fevers. I knew how to help him and after I did, he became an advocate and believed I could help with many things. He came to me after that several times per week working on various health issues. From 2005 until he unexpectedly died in 2010, I helped my dad reverse stage four kidney disease to stage three, with acupuncture and oriental medicine herbal formulas.

My mom had a bone spur and was treated for one year and she never had to have surgery since receiving the treatment. My mom came to me more often also for various reasons. Top of them for lumbar pain due to osteoarthritis. I treated many other ailments and assisted her in keeping her phlegm production down often called accumulations (the body makes them without help) meaning phlegm nodules, cysts, and tumors in Chinese Medicine, as well as her, digestion, immune system and thyroid, function more efficiently. She was required to take a daily formula called Nous, which was known to shrink tumors and provide sustained immunologic energy and longevity to the body. This gave her great energy and brain function, improved immunity, and strength.

I received my board-certified license in 1997, opened my private practice the following year, 1998 and traveled to China to study Advanced Acupuncture Orthopedics. In California, Medical acupuncturists are physicians (e.g., medical doctors, osteopaths, dentists) who have completed additional training in acupuncture.

I have always enjoyed my life and my work. Keeping in mind what is satisfying to me and what I care about, in 2018, I was able to add Reiki training to what I love to bring joy and inspiration to others. I'm inspired to provide Intuitive Acupuncture, advisement, coaching, and consulting to those in and outside of recovery to many aspects of living. What satisfies me deeply is spiritually assisting those who feel they could never be helped. Ones feeling stuck in their job or other areas of life. I've been there, thinking I was trapped, hopeless, doomed, with No Way Out. Many cannot see a way, but I can.

CHAPTER 13

Family Circles

In 2010, acting as a representative and spokesperson for my mother, my sister announced a request to put a feeding tube in my dad, against his legal written wishes. This was the first of innumerable manipulative actions of my siblings over the course of eight years, including manipulation of trust and healthcare power of attorney, impersonating me to the doctor's staff at the hospital.

The events of the past are in the past, and I have been able to forgive all for what was done. It's simple, though not easy. Praying for the willingness to be willing to forgive is where to start. For me, it was many months of daily prayer. The most important factor to remember is *Love no matter what the situation.* In some cases, I have seen healing come full circle within my family.

For nearly thirty years, I spent most Saturday nights going to dinner and a meeting with my dad, as he stayed clean and sober. There are several awesome miracles here. I stayed sober, and so did my dad. We shared a great many special and beautiful moments, one of the greatest of which was being able to share, speak, listen, be heard, and receive his appreciation. He told me that he was very glad he got sober because he was addicted, his hands shook uncontrollably, and it was getting worse. He confided in me that he could only go a few hours without drinking and knew he could not stop on his own.

One of the miracles I did not expect was that he softened up so nicely and became a very thoughtful and kind person. I was able to get my dad back, as I remembered him from my childhood, with his original personality and quick wit dry sense of humor. I will always cherish our Saturday nights together. Just spending time with my stoic dad was a truly beautiful experience, a gift, for which I am in deep gratitude. We shared twenty-nine and ¾ years of sobriety before he passed. My beating heart will always remember how much I loved my dad.

In the year 1992, my mom sat me down and said, *"I would like to thank you for giving me my husband back."* I was impressed, but more so, taken aback, as directly and honestly communicating with me was not what I typically experienced with her. I replied, *"You're welcome. It's a God Shot mom"* and left it at that. This is one of the prime examples of how God has worked through me in my lifetime, unbeknownst to me. I trust that I am needed as God's channel of love, support, and teaching. I can truly see that now.

My mom touched many lives and had hundreds of friends. She had been the main hub and center of attempting to balance the rings of the ism in alcoholism. Possessed by the idea that the future and present happiness can be based upon forgetfulness of the past, she created her new reality by controlling her thoughts. The way she cared for her home, nurturing the many species of orchids grown in the greenhouse by my dad and the beautiful plants were part of her rituals for creating her life as she imagined it. The nightly two cocktails were part of her ritual.

Beginning before my father's death and lasting until the death of my mom, my siblings increasingly interfered with the well-being of our mother and father, as well as in my caring for them in a series of ongoing manipulation, lies, and greed. Upon their clinical interference, they used her surgery recovery to attempt to declare her incompetent, and I was blocked from seeing my own mother. I was videotaped carrying out boxes and falsely accused of stealing. The locks were changed on the house door, and siblings sent a text to me and all relatives stating that they were taking good care of her. In reality, they were touting her to many doctors, in order to get a diagnosis of incapacity. The motive was money and my mother's demise.

My mother fell prey to their tactics, but I saw their agenda and knew it was going to be done in a passive-aggressive manner that my mom would never know. The deeper their controlling and manipulation became, the keener my intuition grew and that guitar string turned tighter in my stomach. I knew deep down inside my mom was in trouble. They were going to mistreat her. They were going to kill her, break her spirit over time. I felt incredibly helpless, powerless, and sad.

My close friend wrote to me; "If I may say, I think it was that your mom didn't have the spiritual ability to fight the others. As messed up as it was, they were her kids too, and when she was 91 years old they suddenly were back in her life frequently for the first time in a long time. And she was glad to have them back. It doesn't mean she didn't love you to the best of her ability. I saw her with you many times and she did love you with all her heart–she just didn't know how to show that to your siblings."

I had cared for my mom's health and well-being over several decades, though none of my siblings knew. They were surprised to find out. They still viewed me as the weak little sister who knew nothing. Despite this, my mom had to protect herself, because of what she created, and as a result, I was the one forced to be outcast by her and betrayed by siblings. There was no other way for her to survive the power of the passive-aggressive trauma perpetrators she had created—*opposing forces fighting over one another over her money*—and she became caught in her own web. Strangely, this pleased her.

The whole situation was quite painful for me to endure. Through working my recovery program, I had developed a clear vision to see all sides of the situation. I was able to step back with unconditional love and understanding of a very complicated situation and circumstance—*one I would not wish upon anyone.*

The part that hurt the most was my coming to realize I loved my mom so much I became co dependent, a warped sense of responsibility I had to let go of. I have come to terms with this and understand my role and my place. This was a long and arduous road to walk, with much dismay and discomfort. Through all of my healing, I became enlightened, and in the evolution of my soul, I understood from her childhood upbringing that she was also traumatized many ways.

With that understanding also came my first awareness of the purpose of my life is to bring joyful evolution and inspiration to others through my experience. To be an uplifter. I was able to bring the gift of learning to love myself full circle, back to my mom. I gave her unconditional love.

During her last five years, we became very close and softened with one another. I regularly went with her to the market to pick out her six-pack of wine bottles, her emollient to soothe her nerves and help her feel like everything is beautiful. She would sit in her chair and look out at the Jacuzzi, staring with delight at the calm clear water. I appreciated so many warm and loving exchanges with her and listening to her positive thinking. I came to finally understand what she had meant all those years when she told me, *"There is a way."* I was able to appreciate for the first time receiving *As A Man Thinketh* by James Allen and the books and pamphlets she had given me, though back then, I could never figure out how to keep the mental thoughts he talked about. I knew how she felt about herself and her own visions. My mom established the reality she desired and knew how to do this. She was natural at creating her own desires. Mom knew how to manifest. She told me that she wanted to live a bit longer.

I am so grateful and appreciative to her for hanging with me for those super tough drinking years. I had several incidents happen over the last of my college years. A series of incidents including traveling across the country with a girlfriend as a passenger totaling her car. Getting the car fixed then driving the highway through the next cloudy, very eerie sunset in Nebraska suddenly hitting a doe and totaling the car. Flying to Chicago finding an infested animal: bugs, roaches all over the mattress carpet and cupboards disgusting eerie unreasonable apartment we rented. I gave up on the experi-ence and the very next night I flew home unexpectantly, feeling like a failure and crowding mom's summer plans. The next fall I became a student out of housing my senior year and stated I was giving up on my college degree. Later finding out it was a breached landlord independent roommate contract. Still, mom believed in me. Mom spent countless days with me, as her using cantankerous teenage daughter searching for housing in Isla Vista. With 200 students out of housing, that year mom stuck to the fact we would find a home for me in Isla Vista. She used the power of her mind. It worked. She met a lady in a bar and found the apartment for me.

After college I had become sober, clean, and clear, I was able to show my mom, unconditional love, for as long as I physically could. She made her transition on July 13, 2017.

In other relationships, the circle of healing in my family has not completed. After my father and I did an intervention on another sibling, who elected to not enter hospitalization.

Years and years after the incident with my sister's husband when I was in college, I brought it up with my well know family therapist. Later, the subject unexpectedly came up in therapy with my sister during her session with the same therapist. Apparently, the therapist broke our confidentiality agreement and told my sister that her husband was not such a good guy. I was devastated. My mistakes became known and talked about, and I came up against further humiliation by my nuclear family affected by alcoholism. My therapist insisted not my fault, however, for that time period, I bore all the judgment and scornful looks rocketed out to me, all of which felt more crippling than my original sin.

Despite the proposed effect on me, I chose not to succumb to running away, or hiding in a drink, pill, or fix. I worked my spiritual program with my sponsor and recovery family. I pressed hard against my Higher Power, my Creator, the people in the program, and my self-help tribes to maintain myself through a power greater than I. I also chose not to retaliate against her.

Her actions showed me that she was not free and, in the moment of witnessing that, clarified to me with crystal clarity the true gift of freedom that came from staying clean, working the recovery steps, and seeing my growth from it. I forgave her and remained standing, holding myself up.

After thirty-plus years of sobriety, using open and honest communication with emotionally mature adults, it was a shock to discover that my siblings were still carrying resentment toward me for my drunkenness nearly three-four decades earlier. Most adult siblings would use a different tactic of communication to work out differences, rather than trickery, slander, severe cruelty, and war that lands in court. The loud outbursts, false accusations, and immature behavior unexpectedly brought back the extreme self-loathing I had developed as a child, as a result of being the scapegoat for ongoing severe and cruel acts. After thirty-plus years of self-growth, I found none of my siblings had grown up. I had no idea how to deal with the reality that someone could stay the same, emotionally, for almost four decades. It was beyond my comprehension and, clearly, outside the capabilities of my spiritual toolbox at that time. Professional trauma therapy became very helpful for me, my powerlessness was brought to my attention and I had PTSD. After a year or more of continued healing, I could understand with much greater sympathy in my heart than ever before in my life. And I could forgive them. Alcoholism affects ALL family members.

In both my family and my husband's family, I recognize the indirect communication, passive denial of truth, and passive-aggressive behavior as the qualifying elements of adult children of alcoholics and codependency programs. In 2018, my husband's oldest daughter was hosting a week-long party in Lake Tahoe for the youngest daughter's fortieth. I had not often attended prior events, but my husband requested my presence at this event honoring his youngest daughter, whom I love and helped to raise since age thirteen. We arrived at the beginning of the week fun festivities and stayed in a home with the boyfriend's two bulldogs and a fourteen-year-old black Labrador, who had a history of hyperactivity as a puppy. The family had been raised in an alcoholic home.

Though they were unable to communicate much with me during our stay, due to dysfunction, I always gave unconditional love and acceptance. So, I did not keep track of the specific behaviors, activities, or drinking each and every day. With that said, the fun times were all drinking events—the all-day drinking at the beach event, the all-night drinking and dancing event, the dinner and cake drinking event, and more. One night, each person picked a song they liked on YouTube and played the music. This was pleasant and required numerous beers and recognition of peers that they know in the recovery program. We all had fun. It was an interesting event.

My husband believes that my siblings must be atheists, because there are miracles all around them, and they literally cannot see them. He is right. They are atheists, in nature, thinking, and manner. I send love as that is the only answer, love, and tolerance.

The children of all my siblings have also been treated with cruelty. This is also, unfortunately, a fact due to alcoholism and our family effects. I personally wanted to stop this. When my son, was young, I refused to let him spend alone time with his grandparents. He got to see them when I was present and around groups, etc. He was raised with unconditional love, structure, recovery principles, and church. As he grew up, I made sure he was not alone for long periods of time and was determined to protect him, at all costs, from sudden insults, barbs, and the like. In later years, I was less protective of my son around my parents as they softened through age and the program of recovery.

Alternatives to recovery may work for other people. I do not want those qualities. I prefer the honesty, open-mindedness, and willingness approach, along with upright, sincere, unconditional love and morality. I grew morally by my willingness to face and rectify errors and convert them into assets. Along with positive continuous sobriety that is what working, applying and embodying this particular spiritual program accomplishes. My past became a principal asset. It takes time to grow up, and some people never do. After a few meetings with my certified EMDR therapy psychologist, I found out just how many of these qualities I had, which qualities each of my parents had, and which they did not. I was enlightened.

I used to let other people wield over me. I gave them the power because of my childhood and past. I was raised to do this. As a result, deep down inside I felt partial to blame and ashamed...not entitled or worthy. What is amazing is what happened to me was not right. That part of me that always felt a need to be validated. To be told, yes you were raised in alcoholism. Yes, this is how I was raised and the abuse of power I had endured as a child had never been acknowledged. I had not even acknowledged this myself. I did not understand what was happening that is why I wrote on my pillow.

As a result of my treatment growing up, I needed to see that my perception was an external reflection of my ego, something I learned from my family. True recovery cannot occur without releasing the ego from the work. The ego wants to protect the individual from further abuse, by comparing, competing, and creating enemies, reacting in the form of an opposing force that is equal in intensity. No spiritual growth or development happens under the control of the ego, because the _ego_ is _E_asing _G_od _O_ut; hence the consciousness does not change. When the ego is not involved in recovery, what is left is unconditional love. As I have stated many times its only 12 inches from my head to my heart. One of the many assets I created from my childhood adversity is my belief, energetically, in inclusivity, not exclusivity.

The ism in alcoholism affects all the family members and future generations. If help is not received the toxicity remains inside each and every person and recycles. I was operating as an instrument of Universal Mind, the Mind of God. Working a program was incredibly helpful, generating much more internal peace and understanding around familial circumstances. I saw my Adult Children of Alcoholics tendencies and patterns. I saw my own alcoholism, and I addressed it. I was the initial family member to overcome addiction. I saw my wrongful actions and made all amends where possible. I saw the alcoholism in my dad and other family members. I was the first in the family to speak the truth and do a professional alcoholic intervention on a family member, my father. I changed the whole dynamic of my family. He agreed to seek treatment and actually stayed sober twenty-nine years, nine months, until he passed.

I am a quadruple winner one day at a time; I grew up in an alcoholic home which means I am an adult child of an alcholic, I am a recovered alcoholic forty years, I am married twenty six years to a recovered alcoholic one day at a time. I am a parent of the same. I had numerous opportunities to find my truth and be the light. I broke the cycle of the family addiction circle. I no longer accept the scapegoat or victim role. I am standing up for myself and passing all that I've learned on to my children and whoever is open to receiving it.

Finding Me and Loving Me– The Deepest Hurdle

Before I can heal myself, I must discover who I am—*Know Thyself*—and come to like myself and love myself, flaws and all. Prior to the beginning of my sobriety, I did not like me. I wanted to exit this life. I did not know me, apart from my disease and family conditioning thoughts of me. Therefore, I did not feel there was any purpose for my being alive. From birth, I felt I was tailored, shaped, and formed in a certain way, in order to act and survive in my family as the predetermined scapegoat. Self-put downs, self-effacement, and critical self-thoughts are common in recovery. As such, most of this kind of thinking was on autopilot for me. I was raised to be a people pleaser in an environment in which the focus of the family conversation was rooted in the need to be right, along with other focuses that don't truly matter.

I was told by professional therapists more than once that having both parents professionally diagnosed alcoholic automatically generated a path of change for me. Yet, we do not see that path until we are on it. We do not embrace and change until we are willing and asking. According to Carl Jung, we are run by our subconscious, and we call what happens to us our *fate* because we do not see the underneath, the subconscious.

Change is the only constant and commonality in life. All living organisms continually change, in order to survive and thrive. We in human form shed our cells, our blood changes every four months. Hopefully, we are able to change our thoughts, beliefs, and behaviors in our pursuit of becoming who we desire to be and with that our need to let go of what no longer serves us.

I was always afraid to look at myself until recovery in my twenties. Even then, I could only peek at myself at first. After many discussions with others, I came to see that we have a lot in common. The relationship with self is key to knowing myself, loving myself, valuing myself, and changing myself. I had to remove the lies I had created out of survival and that I had kept telling myself. My limiting beliefs would continue to stop me if I allowed them to. I had to begin to use an earnest-looking glass. I am the only person who can stop myself. Change is the touchstone of growth. "I am free enough to create my own internal bondage." (Ester Hicks)

On my path to discovering who I really am, I made numerous and large changes. I changed residences—over 2586 miles, my career, my body, my health, and my habits. I transformed my thoughts, my mind, my beliefs, my entire life, and my future. Through my willingness, practices, and dedication to self-discovery and healing, I've been able to develop and reinvent my skill set, the way I work, the way I value my abilities, and what I value.

One day at a time, I changed my perception of reality for the better. I know what it is like to be positive and proactive. I put one foot in front of the other. I did the next indicated thing on the calendar. I lived one day at a time. Change is the only way forward.

I know that the continual change in my life was to discover who I am, who I think I am, what I think, what I believe, what I want, and what way I want to do it. This is the process of self-discovery. I was raised with self-loathing, self-criticalness, and self-judgment, so impatience, self-denigration, and perfectionism have been my biggest learning areas. I had to find out who Robin is, not who I'd been taught to believe she is. My focus became the prevention of any negatives in my thinking. Internal positive self-talk was introduced to me, yet it became a roadblock over time. I only knew the concept from the outside. No matter what I did, an internal embodiment was my challenge. I felt the love from others, yet that did not stop the nights of waking with those voices in my head. The critical voices came whether I wanted them to, or not. I was around the environment of recovery people and the energy of love, but I was not able to change my inside until I started writing and learning about myself. Over time, the uncovering, discovering, and discarding, to find my true self, quieted all those voices in my head. I discovered I am worthy, loved, lovable, and important. I also learned that the woman who is still sick is just as important as the woman who is healed.

In my eleventh year of recovery, I noticed the importance of changing how I think. We live in a world created by the mind. I possess the freedom to choose what I think and the words I say to myself. My vibration, my feelings, and the way I feel about myself are of utmost importance in choosing how to treat myself. I choose to treat myself as I would a close friend or child. When I am disappointed, I must not use words that are harsh, as I used to. Over the course of thirty-plus years, my mom gave me plenty of pamphlets, books, and mementos about changing my thinking to change my life. It has taken years and layers for me to overcome the automatic ingrained negative self-talk.

I eventually came to realize that one of my biggest lessons is how to be kind and loving toward myself. In that realization, my day starts with gratitude. I gave myself a daily dose of love and kindness, as I would offer a close friend. Eventually, my thinking became different, but it took lots of practice, focus, and desire to change. Mom may not have been this way when I was young, and I may not have seen it as I grew, but my very first teacher who modeled how to think differently was my mom. She used thought power every day. I spent the most time with my mom. My early years and teenage years.

With newly learned thinking and disciplines came new values. These all developed into a new belief system, from which came spirituality. I do not follow the masses. I never have. My core energy, aka inner being, soul, spirit, or Christ self is different from the masses. I walk to my own beat, my own vibration. The recovery culture and practices have been my home for forty years. Today, I feel comfortable in many different types of groups.

The best way of loving the self is honoring and being true to self. Through my awakening to who I really am, and who I am not, I discovered that I must embrace my individuality, rather than looking at where I don't fit in. When I follow my own energy, I feel how my insides match my outsides. My outer being, aka human, personality, physical being matches my inner being. I feel aligned and in line with who I really am. If I am unhappy, I know that I am not lined up with the truth of my inner being. Can my personality get off course? Yes. It often does, mostly when I am measuring myself beside others. I am an individual positive creation. I must remember my mission, the purpose I chose for coming to this life experience. My mission is not what someone tells me it is.

I have the ability to self-actualize and grow in wisdom daily if I remain willing to follow my own inner guidance system, my intuition. This is God Consciousness. In the past, if my head, mind, or ego tries to take over, and I start second-guessing my inner guidance, by applying logic, things go askew, out of balance, and sometimes into struggle mode.

I learned through twelve steps that I live by the principle of inclusiveness, not exclusiveness. I use conscious appreciation, focus, and intention. At the age of twenty-two, I learned to take what I want, what resonates with my being and leave the rest. How I grow is to take baby steps. As a human, I am a speck of dust in the vast expanse of the Universe. There are over one hundred names for God and over one hundred paths to lead me there. My way or the highway keeps me narrow. I believe in a diversity of open concepts. It is not one or the other. If I do not agree with a certain dogma, I leave it. This is a personal journey for each and every one of us, and every choice I make is and should be, a personal one. I like to use all different tools out of my personal spiritual toolbox that contains different labels, different shapes, and different applications. I can use one tool over another, and perhaps a different tool over time. I might need a special tool for a special time. If it works don't fix it. I am not stuck on one way, one path only. That becomes a self-limiting box for me. I choose to believe in the positive forces of the Universe. I am open and receptive. This is the highest priority.

The more I came to know myself, the more aware I became of what felt good for me. The more I chose actions that felt good to me, the more nourished I felt. The better I felt inside, the abler I was to appreciate. The more my appreciation grew, the deeper my inner love and joy grew. As my love for life grew, and as I treated myself as I wanted to be treated, the abler I was to love myself. Love for self is critical to be happy and inspired. It is an ongoing, daily process that started with creating new behaviors and turning those into new habits.

Learning to love me through which evolved into a desire and ability to help others love themselves and love life. I never realized anything like this was possible.

Loving me = loving other Relationships

CHAPTER 15

Healing Me

Growing up with alcoholism and the associated dysfunction, neglect, and abuse created anger and resentment in me. I had to write to get sober. For years I wrote many fourth steps, spoke with a confidant, and followed specific actions in my spiritual climb. This process in itself is freeing and growing. Many times, just immediate apologies help. My previous habitual behavior of being a pompous ass while drinking paved the way for carrying guilt during my first sober years, until I made initial important direct amends.

Radical emotional changes had to take place over the years for me to become a sober and productive member of society. Working through my perceived fearful situations each day, checking my motives, maintaining self-honesty, being accountable, and taking the right action was part of it, as were honoring my word, learning how to communicate in a new way. The ability to work through feelings is imperative. All of these and other changes began to free me from my self-imposed prison. Self-improvement through healing is the key.

There are four primary elements for healing and many additional supporting ones. My healing started with number one: abstaining from the drink, pill, or fix. Number two, three, and four, in no particular order, are nutrition, mental focus, and spiritual outlook, or—*more accurately termed—inlook*. Both aspects seem to be necessary.

Sometimes throughout the day I must pause take a few minutes to work with my breath, remain God-conscious. I read published material that speaks to just for today. It talks about a quiet half hour all to me. Meditation, I personally need 17 minutes to a half-hour. For me, Saturday mornings can be extended. An added time during the day works too. I pause at night before sleeping. Reading something from "Psalm or I Am" nourishing to the soul before rest. Night meditations after bedtime preparation are very soothing and produce a positive vibration.

I learned that what I think about is of utmost importance, I must pay very close attention to my need to think about what I am thinking about. When I catch myself thinking negatively, which is less than ten percent of the time now, I have stopped myself in the middle of the self-judgmental thought (phrase) and said to self, *"No, this is the way,"* (pointing or looking up), and I rise above. More internal peace is generated by asking my mind to listen to either nothing (a heater, fan or one of the alternative spiritual words I have learned: "I am" Spirit, Life, Joy, Truth, Love, Intelligence. For those who are not higher power centered the big me and the little me. Speaking 'the word" or phrase over and over in a mantra until another word like it enters my mind. These are added any time of day or around normal prayers. Keeping the *Spiritual mind focus* with no waiver.

I must operate in a higher vibration and energy if I want to be successful and aware of a loving magnificent higher self. This means I need to clear my energy field and raise my vibration. For this, I need to drink a lot of water, eat properly, and moved to a purification nutrition-oriented program, way of being or habit. I need to sit and listen to my creator for at least 12-17 minutes daily, to quiet my mind.

I have worked hard with a good friend and many new friends who are healers. It has been quite a transformation for me to be involved with healers. Some of these folks did recovery their own way. I wanted to get off any and all mind-altering chemicals, no matter what. One day at a time, I do the next step on my calendar. I completely surrendered. Beginning sobriety, I turned myself over to a sober advisor. I followed directions from another person. I had to ask a higher power for help numerous times per day, not even knowing what I was praying to. Walking in blind faith, some call it a jumping-off point. First, it's the doorknob, if you have no other belief. Some say no God, only consciousness. I started my alignment with a friendly power greater than myself that I choose to call God. If I stay truly clean the higher consciousness feeling arrives.

I spent a lot of time striving to become that hole in the doughnut. I did the best I could with the tools I had. I functioned in society. I ran myself silly. Unfortunately, I became strong in some areas and seriously out of balance in others. By the time I came to see a real energy worker, I had become someone with a large rich history of better feeling. thinking and being than I had been in over two decades. One of the best parts, no hangovers.

I began examining my reason for living, asking, *"What am I doing here?"* I realized that I was being guided to somehow find out. So, I started becoming conscious of my search, taking one day at a time. Watching. Listening.

I had grown up learning to be a perpetrator-con man. As an older teen and young adult, I did things my way, trying to run the show. Trying to fit the people to do and be what I wanted, I lied and manipulated those around me. This was all the result of receiving and replicating what I called "perpendicular love" from my family. I had learned well. Ironically, my youngest older sister described me as Erica on *All My Children*. This was my mechanism to survive. If I was more bad-ass than you, I would survive. But, in the process of doing this, I kept damaging myself, drinking my own poison.

It required a very strong effort for me to understand how I was raised and what happened. As adult offspring of alcoholics, or addicts or abusers of any kind, we subconsciously recreate our experiences. There is always a mirror reflecting back to us what we are needing to see, understand, and heal because, at some level, it is still within us and creating experiences for us. We call the experience back to ourselves until we get out from under or raise our awareness.

Having reflected on this often and felt this in my own life experience, I know that I create things that are, from my human perspective, in contrast to my false beliefs about myself and my world. I do this for my own learning and awakening. I recognize what I don't want and can therefore know and understand what I do want. Staying focused on the positive. Listening to my innermost self.

However, I couldn't just leave it at understanding or even knowing. If I didn't change my inner thoughts and feelings, everything would keep repeating, and I would be caught in my own merry go round of internal thought patterns, my own cage. This is often called karma, referring to the principle of cause and effect, where one's intent and actions influence or create one's future.

The primary factor in creation is consciousness. If no change or development in consciousness occurs on the inner level, no amount of action will make any difference in my world. I would recreate modified versions of my world or the same thing again and again. I had to recover from my conditioning by releasing false belief systems and change my thoughts and actions. Using this type of moral psychology, I had to grow up and out of this mindset. In doing so, I discovered the truth underlying many of the mysteries and traumas of my life.

My biggest challenge in changing and healing myself is remembering that everything and everyone is operating on a vibrational frequency. Low vibrational frequencies produce low vibrational thoughts. If I want to feel good, I must change my thoughts to those that feel good, because chronic or long-held thoughts turn into solid beliefs. Beliefs create good-feeling or bad-feeling emotions. Bad-feeling emotions create bad-feeling experiences or realities.

From a very young age, I believed that I was adopted, a creation of my own thinking, resulting from not receiving the love and nurturing I needed to feel good and blossom. Coming down with tonsillitis as a chronic condition was reflective of two emotional issues: never having a voice or being validated; and having a low immune system due to my perception of being chronically sad and unloved, which measure a low vibration similar to that of sickness. It was also an unconscious way to get attention. Instilled in me as a child were the old programming and beliefs that I am not good enough (smart enough, quick enough, pretty enough, funny enough, old enough, perceptive enough, wise enough, valuable enough); therefore, my early feeling of I am not worthy of vitality, love, happiness.

In all of these and other experiences of my childhood, was I legitimately wronged? Injured, yes. I do not negate this. Has this been easy to accept? No. Has it been necessary for me to stay clean and sober? Yes. Often things did not turn out my way. Stating who is right and who is wrong is a complete waste of time and energy. I don't try to regulate anyone but myself. What is most important is that we make better moments. I never knew that. I was just looking at the victim's side.

As a young adult, I never wanted to face the possibility that I had a problem. A quote that always resonated with me is: *"I was a sick person trying to get well, not a bad person trying to get good."* When we attempt to admit that we have a problem, because of our conditioned beliefs, we think that we are weak, wrong, and bad. These thoughts, and the feelings they instill block our recovery. If we think of ourselves as bad, we never believe that we can truly become good. Therefore, the healing and recovery are forever on hold, until the problem is reframed in our mind to accurately define the behavior as a disease, rather than a determination of our morality, ability, worthiness, or humanity. On the other end of the stick, if we believe that we should be independent and strong, we fail, because the cause and recovery are a "we" dynamic, not an "I" process. Initially, this warped understanding kept me stuck for quite some time until I understood that I had not created it independently, and I could not heal it alone. Then, I was able to willingly open myself to help and to the "we" process of recovery.

I arrived at a new understanding. It took me years to learn my own part in it and my integrity lesson, working a program, doing what was required, writing my inventory, looking at my part. I asked for forgiveness of myself and others. I said, *"I now release these words out of my being into the Universe and know that I may change my thoughts instantly."* I learned a lot from that expensive and expansive lesson. I have said and done this repeatedly, utilizing the principles of Law of Attraction.

It is suggested that we play the recording *"You are fearfully and wonderfully made"* (Psalm 139:14) and understand what it means to know that my Creator has made me in a wonderful way. It feels foreign at first. The deep, internal, soul issue for me, a woman recovering from many insidious emotional traumas, was that I just didn't believe that at the time.

Over the years, recovery people would speak from the podium about how we must live (act) our way into right thinking, instead of thinking our way into right living. I've done both. Either way, I think in positive cognitions. Take the slow road or the fast road. I took the slow road. Either way, I can't see until I can see.

My healing has been a long ride—*forty years at the time of this book's publishing*—and expensive. I have elected many forms of healing, even paying a spiritual counselor to tell me what I didn't see. There are many avenues of people to go to for help. The key is finding an authentic person you resonate with who has been born or developed the gift over time by allowing their vibration to rise.

A friend I met in 1980 was trying to show me that meditation is the way to peace and happiness within. I did not take heed at that moment and did not realize that for the ten years from 1980 to 1990, I had been running in a meditative mantra trance. Without my knowing, this helped me change from within. I got rid of my old ideas, moving into emotional sobriety. I have long since integrated daily meditation into my morning routine and feel so much better.

I learned that I need to be positive. However, this positivity must not only be mentally understood, or forced, or even attempted, but fully integrated into me and embodied by me, through my concerted focus on creating this embodiment, thereby changing myself. The more I understand the truth that I am an energetic or spiritual being having a human experience here on earth, the easier it is to stay grounded when the turbulence of emotion or conflict begins.

You may be thinking, *That's fine for you, but I have this problem.* Guess what? The same principle works if I am worried about my dad's drinking, someone else's using or dealing. I may hold them in the palm of God's hand. Picture protection for them. I did this with my son when he lived in Spain for years. I held him in the palm of God's hands. I ask for protection for him. I know he is protected then. I trust in God (Higher Power) clean house, (my own mental emotional spiritual house) work with others (help someone who has less experience than I)

Each one of us has a soul journey. I may be able to support you in your journey however; I cannot change your journey or what your soul has decided it needs in this life. So, I must detach. The meaning of detachment, according to Webster's Dictionary is *objectivity, open-mindedness, neutrality.* I like all three. Detachment leads me away from focusing on the contrast. Nonjudgment. I can raise my vibration for myself. I do not have to be gravely affected by another's opinion or actions, even relatives, close friends, or spouses. Detachment is a release from a desired outcome or control. Consequently, detachment is a release from suffering, as in the Baha'i Faith, Buddhism, Hinduism, Jainism, Stoicism, and Taoism. I use detachment as a spiritual principle. Thus creating the ability to stand up for myself.

Shifting and clearing occur in layers, to the extent of our conditioning and forgetting from birth the truth of who we are. It is a lifelong process that continually unfolds, peels the layers, reveals deeper false beliefs. Of course, this depends on the level of suppression and faulty conditioning of the individual. In my case, it was pretty deep and long, and complicated by the physical effects of the initial substance abuse damage.

As of the date of this book's publishing, I have spent every day of forty years actively and consciously connecting and aligning with my Creator-Higher Power, shifting my thoughts, beliefs, perceptions, and actions for clarity—removing my mental box or shackles, climbing out, and opening and allowing myself to SEE the true source entity energy being I am.

My recovery has been cumulative and expanding awakening, from an eclectic array of clean housework with others, trust in Creator, along with educational enlightenment and learning modalities, experiences, and practices, including; Kundalini meditation, Esther Hicks and the Law of Attraction, listening to inspirational speakers for fifteen minutes daily, and all forms of spiritual healing. I have had the fortunate assistance of all Spiritual Guides. I was introduced to Eastern thought when studying Chinese medicine. This has helped my inner being a great deal because as I mentioned, brought the Twelve Step philosophy with me upon entering the Chinese medicine school. I learned the Chinese philosophy of treating everyone as if I would treat my mom. in 2018,

I began adding the Reiki 5 Elements of Love, Truth, Honor, Gratitude (Appreciation), and Kindness to my chakra balancing.

My parents raised us with all western drugs and medicines. I used to take many over the counter meds. My mom loved the large white pill called Vanquish, her go-to product if she did not feel well, even emotionally. For forty years, I have lived free from reliance on my old beliefs, behaviors, or drugs of most kinds—I strive for no mind-altering chemicals whatsoever—including prescribed drugs. I do take Ibuprofen when necessary. Living life on life's terms, I use no buffers, no soothers, no alcohol. I've even thrown away prescribed drugs. Ibuprofen is the strongest drug I take and not often usually. I needed drugs less than a handful of times in my life due to some surgical procedures, or surgeries. Most dental procedures do not require more than a few hours of meds if any now. Usually, ibuprofen does the trick. I care about the way I feel.

In some circles, alternative pain relievers are fine. I use herbal medicine, oils, and other energetic forms of relief. There are plenty of choices to support the body in feeling good. I now use applied clinical nutrition and ask an expert for help. I utilize all forms of spiritual healing. Improving my thoughts was just as vital as much as any physical pain needing to be addressed.

I was introduced to Eastern thought when studying Chinese medicine. This has helped my inner being a great deal because, as I mentioned, I entered the Chinese Medicine school with my understanding and use of the recovery program philosophy.

I started my journey of Chakra energy healing. My Chakras were so off-balance as I did not know my true energetic self. If I am not in balance spiritually, things are produced out of my wishes because I am holding the wrong mental focus. If my mental focus is not aligned, then I travel a road I do not wish to go down I find myself seeing this later after traveling that road. If I stay grounded and keep my chakra energy centers in alignment, I can soar.

Shaman healing was a significant day for me. I was referred to a disciple of John of God, a disciple of the well-known greatest healers in the world. After driving from Orange County to the Los Angeles hills area, I knocked on the door at 10:38 am. After waiting a few minutes, I noticed that the energy vibration from the ground and all around me was very high. I felt so warm. As I filled out a questionnaire in her living room, she asked me some questions about how I felt and what I needed. I answered that I had a hesitancy and low-level anxiety inside, despite doing everything I could think of to help it, including seeing a sound healer who helped to balance and clear chakras for me, which helped me feel better, but I was still stuck. I explained that I felt remnants I could not understand or heal myself with, through the previous many various levels of healing over the last thirty-seven years. I told her about the eye desensitization therapy healing I received from the psychologist for my trauma-induced PTSD. She stated that he helped me. I explained about my childhood and emotional trauma from my upbringing. I shared that my deepest desire was to be free from my trauma. I wanted to be free.

I soon found out what type of gifts she had. During a near three hour energetic procedure, I watched my spirit guide leave me to be with this healer and assist. I felt dozens of others aiding my shaman. The experience was amazing. In the end, she told me, *"You did not have a choice about what happened to you as a child. You signed up to be in this role in this life to teach the others about their lessons."*

In May 2019, I cleared a new layer. Until now, what has gotten in the way is my underlying consciousness, operating by default, without my awareness. I asked for help, and today I received it—clarity, awareness of what had previously been blocked from my sight. I had been hiding, because, subconsciously, I made myself not belong. After all, I was branded the black sheep, the scapegoat. As such, I subconsciously self spoke in a way to make myself not belong, a ruling of myself that I developed in the beginning as a child. Therefore, I didn't fit, and I was not rejected, so I was safe.

Some call this a pattern. I could not see it before, and I am genuinely grateful to the woman who did. It was during the process of writing this book that I realized that I was subconsciously re-experiencing a toxic memory of being disregarded, neglected, overtly criticized, unloved, ashamed, and rejected. I had the clarity

I was subconsciously creating this pattern and to clear the lingering wreckage from my past. The neural circuits had been identified and rewired.

The deep-rooted beliefs, behaviors, and habits remain until I make a decision for the clarity to change them. It's a decision to change, to be in alignment with God's view of me, and embodiment by footwork. Prayer and action, *Treat and move your feet.* It is a God consciousness moment to moment decision to change, followed by moment to moment footwork.

Self-love, self-knowledge, and self forgiveness are always the keys to releasing the negative self-thoughts and feelings we were conditioned to. Embodying new beliefs about ourselves and others and new principles to live by is necessary if we are to change what we hand down to our children and future generations. I had to ask myself, *"What values am I really delivering?"* Monkey see monkey do shifts in each and every moment from this new clarity. I had to change my monkey habits for my survival, as well as for the benefit of self and others. I am available to my children when they call. I am available to help other people when they call or text nowdays. That is how I remain of maximum service, to myself, to my God, to my fellows.

I learned that I must continually be willing and teachable. Becoming clean, clear, conscious, and connected is a life-long process. I grew up starting with the prayers listed in the recovery bible as I call it. I still say them today. I love the openness and inclusiveness and the spiritual principles, which—when properly embodied—create lasting peace within. I must continually be committed to my ongoing health and healing, through using whatever methods and tools I'm inspired to use at the moment.

Above all, I had to learn that my thoughts and vibration are my priority. From committing to these, no matter what others do or say, my personal energy is no longer affected by others. Years ago, I began exchanging those negative self-thoughts with new positive self-words that bring myself congruent with God's view of me. Why be incongruent, out of alignment with my true Source made self? If I do, I am just stopping myself by listening to the old talk.

I position myself as the third-party observer and instantly replace those words. I line my mind up with Source, while simultaneously not produce conflicting thoughts as I'm stopping the forward momentum with the incongruent self-talk. If I hold two opposing thoughts at the same time—one aligned and one incongruent—I am giving myself a double message and holding split energy, which just takes me spinning. I must stay in the now. If I have one foot in tomorrow and one in yesterday, I will urinate all over today. I must hold the message of the one aligned positive thought and stay clear.

So, I send the negative thought away at that very moment and replace it with one of the words or phrases I learned in Reiki entrainment teaching, aka a Spiritual Principle. I focus on that word or phrase and do not wobble or stray. I stay focused on it for sixteen or seventeen seconds. This is coupled with a Five-Element application. If I can focus on it for another seventeen seconds, I do. This continues until my mind becomes stronger, tuned in, and inspired and produces another word or phrase. As I do this, I line up with God's view of me, my spiritual energy shifts, and my vibration rises. I must target as the third observer and instantly replace those words. I am a locomotive, a rocket, my intention is in gear, and forward motion must occur. I become my own observer.

With all of this said, it is most important to be always authentic and humble and to know that as we shed old skin that no longer fits us, the newly revealed skin underneath is fragile and newborn. We will experience the fear and the slips and wonder if we have forgotten everything we have learned and integrated. All is not lost. Recovery, self-discovery and healing are a lifelong cycle that happens in layers. We move to deeper levels and get to apply principles in a new way to the new layer.

I was raised with, required to learn, and operated in a lot of self-denigration. Newly sober, I walked around with the negative self-talk for years. After forty years of working on myself, it occasionally happens that if I feel I have made a huge mistake, I automatically move into self-denigration. It is a default habit that, though lessening and healing, is always ready to shift back into autopilot, taking me with it. Usually dormant, up till now it would suddenly rise, unexpectedly offering me an opportunity to apply all of my work and reprogramming at a deeper level.

Up until now, I have gone along, accepting that I do or think in certain ways. I ask Christ,Spirit and God to remove this, as I toss out old ways. I wonder how in the world I would begin to change it. I have read books and listened to people who advise me in ways I need to think and treat myself. Spiritual Mind treatment and spiritual energy treatments are a way.

What I have learned in recovery is we strive to get better through the right action. Generally, this leads to the goal of right thinking. However, I must erase the negative by iterating and reiterating something positive. If I allow the negative thought or feeling, I erase it as soon as I am aware, and I reiterate the new truth I know. It takes time. I must check in with the feeling. I ask myself which statement feels better to me and which is more congruent with my Creator's view of me and my purpose here on earth. Gratitude is always a better feeling. Along with Jesus Christ and the Angels at my side, I employ daily Reiki, meditation, Qi Gong, and super thought powers to move upward and forward.

Everyone has multiple and different ways they communicate and receive guidance. Throughout the forty years of my new life, I have had a need to commune with different entities at different times, for different circumstances and my alignment. I have changed over time. Every morning, before I speak to anyone, I spend time with the Lord, aka my Higher Power, God, Source, Spirit, Jesus, Buddha, my Creator, Kuanyin, my Angels and Guides. I pray and have access to all of these entities. The only door which needs to open is mine. I changed my behavior from jumping out of bed onto the earth as a human, to taking baby steps from my Spirit-connected state, meditating in a sleep-like state, especially the first seventeen seconds upon awakening. This is crucial to set my vibration and connection for the entire day. This is my new entrainment. I set my intention, consistently aligned with the light, and ask for sobriety, divine guidance, right thinking, and appreciativeness.

In the past, I woke up in the middle of the night. I could not sleep. I had too much on my mind, not living in the present. This has happened a lot since late 2016, not sleeping. It was a temporary pattern. I lay in bed, tossing and turning, as my mind kept gyrating. I practiced breathing techniques. I told myself to be quiet and focus only on one thing to keep a quiet mind. But the mind would not stop thinking. I knew I had to write.

I had something to write about. As I did since I was a child. I began to write, though no longer on my pillow. As soon as I write, my mind quiets again. Why? I have freed my mind from disturbing me with the feeling, and I have created a feeling through written expression I can reference again when I need to. At that point, I am free to *Let go and let God*. This is trust in the universe issue. I must trust. Just Trust. If it's in the past, I write and let go. If it's in the future, I put it in the God jar and let go. I let go.

There are various tools I use to pray to my higher self and open my communication. One is a five-step prayer learned nearly thirty-nine years ago through the study and use of Science of Mind classes and principles. Most recently, I have employed entrainment through my hands to myself, for energy balancing and thought pattern change. It is used in the Master of Circadian Rhythm. I concentrate and hold the light and hand energy to myself. Many days have been more positive and peaceful for me because of the training. Many nights have been more restful.

Still, this is a world of contrast and cycles. Just a few days ago, I mentally slipped and caught myself. I was mad at myself and could not identify how or why I switched from love and acceptance for myself to downright screaming at myself for my mistake. I went to the LA County Records to pick up my mother's death certificate and my birth certificate. The wait in line was forty-five minutes. The people were nice and friendly. After waiting, I had to leave to get the appointment letter at home to prove that I needed an emergency copy of my birth certificate and return the next day. I then had to return a third time to pick up my birth certificate. I had placed the payment receipt in a plastic sleeve to keep the paper protected. In the parking lot on the way in, I was stopped by a sales-person. Somehow, while talking with him, the receipt slipped out without my knowing. When I got home, I actually threw my purse and screamed at myself, *"You _____! How could you do this!?"* I realized my childhood memories of how I was being talked to and that my diseased alcohol abusive inner self-talk had shifted into autopilot and taken out my mental whip. I was genuinely upset with myself to my core. A few minutes later I realized what I had said to myself and thought, *I need to still work on me. What triggered me to get so mad at myself for the mistake?* I then imagined not being able to get my certificate and asked myself *What's the worst thing that could happen?* I could stand in line and reorder.

I am not alone if I act to help myself. Even devastated, I have a choice to do something to help pick myself up. When I asked to feel better, I was led to recovery and support, as God put the right people in my life at the exact moment and place, I needed them. I still work on my self-development day by day, by recognizing, releasing, and asking myself for forgiveness at that moment. This is one of the processes that enable me to change, the awareness of my thoughts and where they go. If I allow indolence, brutality, confusion, impurity, and corruption in my thoughts, my feelings become depressed, and my vibration descends. I will block my change and healing if I have a poor mental attitude of *What's the use?*

I am human. I know today I absolutely do not want negativity in my energy vortex and ask this to be removed. I never give up on myself. We live in a mental world. My mom taught me to keep my hand firmly on the helm of thought. I must become aware of a thought and take the right mental action. Awareness is forming a new mental attitude. Having my observer out helps to monitor my own thinking, so I always remain aware and uplifted. I know what is right. I have a prominent Master who is awake inside my soul. Self-control, right thought, peace, and calmness. This makes vibration ascend.

I have traveled many paths of healing myself over the forty years since first becoming sober. Through new people and a new family, I have truly had twelve kinds of healing. Here is a timeline of most of the modalities I employed along my journey.

- 1980 Sudden Psychic Change (Spiritual Experience) facilitated Sobriety; Reading *Just For Today;* Attending Unity and Science of Mind Spiritual Centers; Daily Writing and Gratitude

- 1981 Psycho Therapy Family Recovery (father); Faith in Higher Power; Structure; Exercise (running) Sober and Single

- 1982 Setting Goals; Twelve Step Recovery Methods to Daily Life; Changing My Thinking

- 1983 Being of Service; Spiritual Devotion; Spiritual Angelic Healing

- 1980-1986 Workshops; Motivational Seminars;

Audiotapes; Nature submersion/Earthing; Hatha Yoga; Controlled Breathwork

- 1987 ACA (Adult Children of Alcoholics) Professional Therapy

- 1988 Science of Mind Training Center for Spiritual Living Riverside, CA

- 1990 Chiropractic Care; Nutritional Healing; Physical Self-Care; Diet; Self-Love; *Emotional Sobriety*

- 1991 Traditional Chinese Medicine; Acupuncture College (Healing Methods,Philosophy)

- 1992 Meditation; Qi gong

- 1998 Learning and Applying New Methods Eastern Medicine Orthopedics and Traumatology

- 2003 Studied Doctor of Naturology Program at AIHT

- 2010 Chakra Healing

- 2012 Developing My gift–Spirit Guide Cognition; Asking for Guidance-Allowing-Following; Abraham Hicks/Law of Attraction/Vibration & Emotional Frequency. Spiritual Writing applications

- 2016 EMDR Emotional Trauma Therapy (Eye Movement Desensitization & Reprocessing); EFT/Tapping (Emotional Freedom Technique); Newer Yoga practices

- 2017 Baptism; Reiki Training

- 2018 Shaman Healing; (Receiving) Kundalini; Daily Meditation
- 2019 Spiritual Healing; Training and Receiving

We all have resources. It's just a matter of changing our perspective so that we can become aware, notice, develop, and earnestly practice until embodied. I reach into my spiritual toolbox. This toolbox really grows and changes over time. I may add more tools as I work with others, learn, and apply what I've learned.

The greatest discovery in my healing, self-development, and spiritual awakening is that I decided on this path for my own expansive and enriching experience on earth. I am blessed to have found myself, learned to love myself, and discovered how to align my body, emotions, thoughts, and actions with the light and love of God. Alchemy.

CHAPTER 16

Understanding My Gift

When I became an adult, I finally understood what my mom meant when she told me that I was special, and ....in my mid-twenties I met a recovery friend in Florida who loved to seek out spiritual healers. When I visited one night at her home. I noticed energetic movements in her kitchen. I was nervous and a little frightened, slightly confused and unsure. When I walked around her living room, I felt the pressure and said excuse me because I could feel strong density of a body yet I could see nothing at the time. I sat back on the couch where I felt I was safer. I did not understand this type of knowing.

151

I never remembered I saw or felt anything at my home, therefore, this adventure was at first clearly foreign to me.

As a Source created a being, I am energy in movement, continually operating through vibration. In having this temporary human experience, with the adversity, lessons, and earthly circumstances—including being conditioned by my family and environment—my senses had become dimmed and less acute, thereby lowering my vibration. If an angel or spirit guide is communicating with me, or guiding me, I must allow my vibration to rise, in order to feel them and even more to see them. Most of us rarely see them, because they are on a different vibrational frequency than we are, a different radio station, so to speak.

The more clean, clear, conscious, and connected, the more my vibration began to rise, I began seeing what I would describe as light bodies or the faces of my spiritual guides and others above me, in the mirror, and in the windows. I did not know who they were, and I could not understand why.

I felt a presence in my office as well. I felt guidance directing me where to place the acupuncture needle, outside of the prescription I had previously decided. The client was significantly better because of it. I usually followed my prescription, however, I began asking for guidance while I work, knowing the information is coming from higher wisdom than my human knowledge.

The reason we need to think positive and feel positive has to do with allowing our vibration to rise. I learned lumens are vibration work, and the frequency is the number of cycles of energy vibration we operate at per second. Angels and other light beings operate at a much higher vibration than humans.

I asked God, Jesus, for this knowing. This ability to be intuitive.

CHAPTER 17

For the Readers:
A Guide to Self-Healing
and Life Balance

It does not matter whether you are an addict, depressant, or abuser, whether you are from Park Avenue or a park bench, or whether you are a surgeon, pastor, movie star, priest or street bum. Deciding to become sober,clean and clear is not a joke. It is life or death. There is no halfway. The statistics are one out of ten succeed at staying clean consistently and persistently. It does not matter the source of the chemical. Alcohol and drugs and perhaps some foods are mind, body, spirit-altering chemicals.

Quickly running from diagnosis to diagnosis is not the answer. Becoming and remaining clean and clear is not about seeking knowledge to control drinking. Covering with chemicals, no matter where they come from does not give the body or mind or spirit an honest chance. Staying purely clean is the answer. Willingness to go to any lengths to achieve sobriety for twenty-four hours, one day at a time, is the requirement.

The primary reason for the failure of the user, abuser, or depressant is the thought, *my case is different*. They must take action that they do not yet believe in. In all cases, it's a matter of limited and illusionary perception. True, lasting recovery and healing can be attained through many paths, as shown in my own forty years of healing and awakening. The purpose of any true recovery program is to stay sober and change one's falsely perceived reality. Following the recommended methods, steps, and tools will save your life.

To begin recovery, the first step is the hardest. The individual is loaded with false assumptions, one of which is that he can cut down and slowly stop. The sunlight of the spirit cannot reach a chemical-filled body. One of the most helpful and true pieces of guidance given to me was, *"Start right where you are, and come to believe that it is possible, starting right where you are—no matter who you are, how you are, or where you are."* Dive into recovery. Don't cover it up. One cannot access what your Creator has intended for your inner being if chemicals are blocking the light of the Spirit.

There are many methods to overcome addiction, including doing it on one's own, shock therapy, aversion or variances of it, hypnosis, inpatient or outpatient centers for alcoholism, Twelve Steps, Twelve steps with Christ, meditation without Twelve Steps, positive thinking, or other therapies. Only from my experience, the main difference between those and the Big Book of Twelve Steps with spiritual actions is that other therapies potentially leave the person in arrested development. I am referring to page fifty-one of Ernest Hemingway's use of the term in *The Sun Also Rises*. Or, mental status develops in other ways. If there is no transitional recovery therapy for the individual to integrate back into society, the development will be arrested.

Alcoholism affects the whole family, not just the person using it. If others are left without the help of mental-emotional spiritual tools, they too remain in arrested development. The disease is just that—a dis-ease, missing ease in life, an imbalance. True healing includes a daily moral inventory, not a one-time treatment, not a one time analysis. The daily spiritual condition, utilizing spiritual applications in proper order is what worked in making my psychic change. I watched it happen inside me, and I witnessed a profound psychic change in countless others over the past forty years. In fact, according to my therapist at the time, anyone may utilize, apply the twelve steps they don't even need to be affected by alcoholism.

Some get off drugs or booze without a program. Yet, they still work in a bar or are around the booze. One thing I learned the hard way is to remove the geographic element related to my addiction, going back to my parents and looking to them for support. I grew up in an alcoholic home and tried to get sober within a practicing alcoholic home. As a recovery advocate, I know that going to the wrong source for what is needed is a big step to learn, looking at the source one chooses for help. I did not know about choosing the right source until I was offered the chance to repeat the step. Looking at, working in, or going to the wrong source are easy mistakes to make. As my advisor told me, *"Do not go to the hardware store for bread. A diabetic does not regularly visit a candy store."*

Going to the correct human source is vital for anyone and for survival and staying clean and clear. Going straight to the Source is direct. Listening to what my Creator, God, Source, Inner Spirit, Higher Power, Angels, and Guides—whatever you want to call it— is communicating and giving to me the answer. I can interpret my higher power as *The Big Me,* or I can follow a doorknob. It really makes no difference. The intention to be clean, clear, conscious, and connected is the key. See how the body, mind, and spirit can heal. Give all three a chance.

To become clean, clear, conscious, and connected, structure is desperately needed. More often than not, there is no structure in the addicted person's life. By age twenty-two, I had none in my life, because I created that. My own series of decisions and desires led me to be alone. When alone with no structure, the afflicted using his certain or uncertain judgment and repeats the random behavior that results in seeking immediate and instant gratification. Successful sobriety requires the whole person, flaws and all, to be right here and right now in all body sounds, emotions, and thoughts. Having structure, including routine habits, prayer, acting my way into right thinking, and just showing up then allows the archetype to take over and a psychic change to occur, thereby creating transcendence.

Remain willing and open-hearted, employing courage, belief, and acceptance. For successful rehabilitation that lasts, stringent honesty, humility, appreciation, and the release of self-centeredness are required, along with gratitude, unselfish service, and faith. One must be fearless in the practice of faith. Working the spiritual path as quickly as possible may just be a fine answer.

If there is previous trauma of any type, it must be removed. If I am enlightened but miserable, the problem is at the core of my soul and thought process. My inner-thinking needs to change. As a child, I was programmed for negativity, growing up in alcoholism and critical parenting. My parents were the critics, and I had five of them—two sisters, one brother, my mother, and my father—all telling me what to do. Internal childhood programming can take as much time to change as I took to create it and as much time as one is willing to prioritize it. To this day I need someone to help remind me to continue my change in thinking. This comes in many forms and applications. Many times, if negative thoughts arise I need help.

When I do, I'm in contrast to what my higher power, my Creator, knows and feels about me, so I feel uncomfortable. In discord, my body starts to decline. I might get a cold, a headache, or bring some unwanted pain, person, or circumstance into my experience. I have free will to create. Therefore, I must instantly shift my thoughts and focus to a higher, more loving one, so I am lined up with Source. To help me see what I'm doing, or not doing. At times, I need feedback from someone, to help me be more aware and stop self-sabotaging and get back on track to my alignment. But, it's imperative to remember that all humans have perception filters that direct their thinking and opinions in ways that may not be helpful. So, why not go to the source?

After I began my recovery, my parents grew and changed also. Yet, even if they never changed or grew, my old programming had to change. If it is going to be, it is up to me. Experience is the component of supreme value in life, particularly if one is willing to turn the past mistakes into beneficial changes. Willingness is a necessary tool. We grow by our willingness to face our false ideas, steps and thinking, rectify them, and convert them into assets. The past thus becomes the main asset, not only of the individual but of the family or group as well. Frequently, it is the domino that paves the way for others in the family or relationships to heal their past and thinking. Sometimes, it is the only asset of the family.

Without tools, assistance, and a willingness to change, it is easy to remain in default patterns of thinking and feeling, aka holding old, learned thinking patterns, beliefs, emotions, and vibrations, due to not knowing what to do, how to improve God-consciousness, or align with Source.

Whether you or someone you know, is in recovery or experiencing another type of crisis or continuing life challenge, it is very helpful to try one thing. Pick one. There are many paths to become more clean, clear, conscious, and connected, all of which allow our vibration to rise

Here are some:

- Do not hold resentment. If you have one, write about it, talk about it, or ask assistance from a licensed person or the silent someone you admire. Any trusted servant will do.
- Stay away from self-pity. Switch your focus on something that you appreciate, that is fun, beautiful, inspiring, uplifting, engaging.
- Remove restlessness. Find a healthy, engaging, fun avenue to move your body and focus your mind.
- Remove irritability and discontent. Get plenty of sleep and

rest. Seek to satisfy your dreams, ideas, and desires. Find avenues of creativity.

* Find someone, a group, or an organization to help. There is always someone you can help.

* Become conscious of your thoughts, words, attention, and feelings. Everything you think, talk about, focus on, believe, and feel becomes your reality.

* Find something that you think is special, delightful, or beautiful, and allow yourself to feel and savor your appreciation of it.

* Be conscious of the foods you eat. Are they dead (packaged, processed, animal), fatty, sugary, doughy, alcohol, or filled with chemicals, hormones, artificial additives, or preservatives? These all bring your energy, emotion, and vibration down (and your weight up).

* Eat fresh fruit. Do a fruit cleanse. The fruit is the highest vibrational food, which helps to detox the mind, body, and spirit.

* Drink purified water—half your body weight in ounces per day.

* Meditate. If you don't know-how, put in some earplugs, close your eyes, and listen to your breath. Keep refocusing on listening to your inhales and exhales.

* Rest and relax every day.

- Get 7-8 hours' sleep every night.

- Midnight to six am on a circadian clock is called Yin within Yin time and is the most inward time and most effective for rest.

- To keep from mental spinning out, thinking about the amount that you must do, employ grounding and balancing techniques to help your roots remain on the earth.

- Walk bare-footed in the grass, earth, and sand.

- Get natural sunlight as often as possible.

- Find animals or pets to watch, listen to, hold, play with.

- Be grateful for every great and small thing and the person you can think of right now.

- Practice acts of kindness.

- Sing out loud.

- Get your blood pumping through some type of movement, dance, exercise, or recreation.

- Find your spiritual belief of choice and connect to it. Even if you don't believe in a higher power, Utililize the Big me and little Me, go on a nature hike, lay in the grass and watch the clouds, swim in the ocean or creek, listen to wildlife, listen to earthlike music, do yoga, or read a spiritual affirmation book.

- Healing the Three Treasures. In traditional Chinese Medicine and Qigong, the practice of healing the three treasures is extremely helpful and very effective. The Taoists believed that one must refine vitality into energy, refine energy into the spirit, and refine spirit into openness. Openness is the place we meet with Source, the place of origins, the place we come into physical beingness from and go back to. These treasures are the energy bases within us: Jing: Essence *or Creative Energy*, Qi: Vitality *or Life Force Energy,* and Shen: Spirit *or Spiritual Energy*. They are vibrational frequencies that interact with and relate directly to our total state of mental, physical, and spiritual well-being. The healing incorporates elements such as movement, power breath, consciousness, thought, and reflection.

If you want to change and realize your dreams to have a life that you desire, the change must begin with you. Quit judging yourself. I cannot explain how to ride a bike. Balance is the key. Seek satisfaction each moment. As an alternative, seek peace. You have a chance, if you are willing to start—somewhere, anywhere, right where you are at this moment. If you do not have the willingness yet, pray for the willingness to be willing until it comes. It will come. When it does, you will gain your clarity and discover the purpose for your time on earth. You must stay on your purpose, even if you fall down, forget, or can only manage one minute at a time. Growing more clean, clear, conscious, and connected is a process. I call *"slobriety"(sobriety)*. Growth takes time. Don't keep track of how much time it takes, only how you feel. One day you will turn around and see how far you've come.

Philosophy for Success

My beliefs become my thoughts
My thoughts become my words
My words become my actions
My actions become my habits
My habits become my values
My values become my destiny

—Mahatma Gandhi

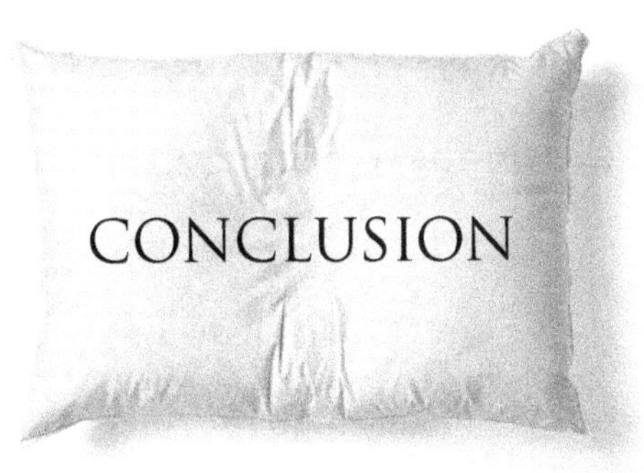

CONCLUSION

Today

When I look back, it seems like a dream. I began this life feeling like I did not fit in anywhere. At a young age and again at twenty-two, I wanted to exit this life. The friend who went with me to Europe for high school graduation is still a good friend of mine. A few close high school friends are still alive, but the serious partiers died a long time ago. How I survived, I don't know. I could have had a nervous breakdown. I could have jumped from the balcony of that building. There were too many forces against me. *There, but for the grace of God go I.*

Recovery defined for the recovering alcoholic is no drug intake, walking clean not only from alcohol and mind-altering drugs but false perception, suppression of feelings. Being successful in recovery is life or death for more than 14,892 days, 40 consecutive and successful years, holding to the twenty-four-hour clock, living each moment in this now-present time, one step at a time. Helping others do the same. (HOW) Honesty open-mindedness, willingness. I began my recovery by noticing, being willing, and learning loving. The toughest being objective third eye self-honesty. Noticing early on that my insides (inner being) and outsides (personality, physicality, expression) did not match. Becoming right sized meaning I am no longer served by feeling better or less than anyone. A feeling of peace within the Universe and connected to all. Being willing to think differently. Learning to align. Loving my insides and seeing their truth. This began as God Consciousness something the Big Blue Book talks about.

I discovered that I do not follow the masses, and never have. I learned that I must embrace my individuality, instead of looking at where I don't fit in. It is not my job to fit in and never was. My whole energetic being is different. I walk to my own beat, my own vibration. This is my energetic being, my Spirit, my God-Christ Consciousness' self. When I follow my energetic being, I feel my insides match my outsides. I feel aligned, lined up. When I'm aligned, I'm aware I always employ honesty and follow my word. If I am unhappy, it is because my personality or expression is not aligned with my energetic being; my G Forces, higher power, Source.

Can my personality get off course? Yes. Sometimes, it is because I am comparing myself, something that was conditioned into my behavior at a very young age. Frequently, I find that I am measuring myself with younger souls who have not learned the same truths as I. I used to believe that, after listening to a positive speaker, my life would change. That did not happen. I went back to my subconscious negative programmed thinking. Nothing changed until I changed the internal negative processing. Making a gratitude list is absolute but my core beliefs and self-conversation had to change also. I'm talking from one microsecond to the next microsecond. I have done this with daily guidance. Action and more Action, as I must employ my daily recovery principles of honesty, open-minded willing (HOW) gratitude, and self-honesty. Something most people are truly unaware of.

If I remain aligned, aware, and willing to receive through learning experiences and follow my own inner guidance system, I grow in wisdom daily. If I second guess my inner guidance system—*my intuition, my energetic vibration*—and force thinking, ego attachment, rationalization, or logic, things go askew, off course, and become sticky, or difficult. If I meditate, things improve.

I found my life work by asking for help from Spiritual healers.

I did not listen at the time and the Universe offered getting rear-ended by a 3M truck. This led me to a physician healer and I found out I had depleted all my physical reserves and to employ big personal daily changes I had to begin the self-love and care program for Robin. This led me to study and become a Licensed Acupuncturist, Oriental Medicine Practitioner in California. I created a very big challenge being in recovery and making it through the coursework because I worked 70 hours a week and traveled for my work.

After all these years I found I like working alone at times and then balancing with others in sharing office space. I use Chakra alignment, Acupuncture and Chinese medicine for longevity, just feeling better myself, and improving my own rejuvenation. I also use whole food nutrition, the body scan muscle test to determine which organs are out of balance. I am a physical movement person and I love applied kinesiology so I am connected with this. I often meditate and then have to move to align with my creator. I successfully do automatic writing to get clear messages.

My lessons are large in this lifetime. I have and will continue to shift and clear what has been handed down to me—the addiction, dysfunction, and recovery on both sides of my ancestry, for generation after generation. I set an intention for it to end with me so that in my generation there will be no more. I wrote on my pillow and repented for my part and my actions. I prayed for self forgiveness. It is important to know my own mistakes and the lessons I learned from them. If I do something to offend someone, I clear up my side of the street and do my part to correct my action idea or disturbance. I invited Christ consciousness into my heart. I initiate change by bringing the issues to the light. I now align myself with Source daily, sometimes moment by moment. With God all things are possible—or for the agnostics, *the Big Me and the little me.* In recovery, the higher power or God is deep within (any name of personal choice).

It's easier to receive the answer when I am in alignment, rather than seeking it from another human. Another human just adds a different interpretation to sift through. Most people attempt to judge looking from their human eyes. Human eyes are limited, even ordained human eyes. I must see clearly without the human body. Today I go directly to the Source, through my inner guidance system, by feeling, perceiving, and spiritually-energetically-intuitively knowing. My own answers will come if my house is in order and dial the right channel. When I do this, my beliefs move from rigid, boxed, and conventional to open, loving, and allowing. When life gets difficult, it helps to remember why I signed up to come to this life, my mission. My mission is not what someone tells me it is. Only I can have an awareness of why I am here. When I ask what is my purpose, I receive the answer. My observer's eye is keen now. I then move in that direction, remain positive, and enjoy each moment.

I originally believed that life happened to me—including being born from my parents and into my family—not knowing that I selected them and generated my challenges for the purpose of awakening to my truth and overcome them.   I know this is true today because I reviewed my own history and tested my own energy center. The way I view or perceive events, people, and occurrences, and where I focus my energy, is what I will receive in return. Most important is to keep an open mind. I see what I am doing now. Through my new sight, I gained the capacity to change and have changed. I practice thinking differently. I send Spiritual healing and loving thoughts to others.

I used to think of the world as so vast and regularly feel overwhelmed by it. Many times, in my sobriety, I arrived at a place where life seemed to have become too big to cope with—the awful, menacing future, that unending nightmare of shadowy days, months, or years! I couldn't even bear to think about it. Well, I quit thinking about it. In reality, life is not too much for me. I do not personally see or interact with its vastness. But life can seem to be too vast around me. When it does, I must get life back into focus. We live in a mental world. I must alter my askew perspective because I have lost the correct one. I regain perspective by applying the right thought and shifting my attention, a split second at a time, one minute at a time, and then one day at a time. I stay inside twenty-four hours. I focus on one thing at a time. I live one breath at a time.

I see, talk, and interact with my own home, my shop, my town, those I live with, work with, assist, and am acquainted with different circles. Circumstances change. My Higher Power concepts remain. I trust, love, and honor, and express gratitude and kindness. I stopped living in a tomorrow that may never come and started living one day at a time—today. I plan for tomorrow, but in my mind, I live only till bedtime tonight. I leave the results up to the Universe.

Today I know that I must follow my dreams. To know their identity, I write, as I did on my pillow growing up. I write down my goal and my name and birth date on the right-hand upper corner. When I write down the goal, dream, or desire, the universe opens and sends me what I desire, according to my vibration. So, I must align my energy first and always! Then, what I dream will come true.

Great events have come to pass for me because of my HP, sober experience strength, hope fellowship on the twenty-four-hour clock. Through my twelve levels of healing and studying forty + years. God willing, forty-one years sobriety on October 8, 2021, God willing. I created a new design for a living. I have made a difference long term, living a life one day at a time, turning over results to power beyond me, being in alignment daily. The results of my soul return allowed me to appreciate me. *My intention and my heart are in the right place today. I am a rock. You can count on me. I believe in my own success. I feel like a gratelful rocket. I am proud of myself.* I am a fabulous product of my life. *I have more to be grateful for today than ever before in my life. I would never trade the experience, faith, growth and the love of my fellow man.*

I am in deep appreciation for the teachers, guides, healers, and meditation facilitators I have met. Caring about how another person is doing is important. Today, I focus on what I can do for another human being. I focus on internal peace. I have evolved and transformed myself into my destiny. I am healthy and abundant. I have become the hole in the doughnut, transformed, evolved, and changed behaviorally, physically, emotionally, spiritually, and in every way possible. I am always a work in progress. People often say that it's an inside job. I know that it's a moment to moment, right now job. We never stop. I am a different person than I was just a few weeks ago. I leave the door open for growth. I remain teachable and changeable.

I have discovered, after all these days, that my disease is a disease of perception. I have been taught how to see and perceive differently. If I am struggling, I have a choice. If I am too stressed or having the feeling everything piling up on me, I ask myself, *"What is important?"* Sometimes, my looking glass is askew. I ask for reality checks from those I appreciate. In addition, Why not go to the Source? It took me a long time to find how to talk to the right source for me. It just takes practice.

The vibration and thought change are what has been most significant to me of late in my healing and movement forward in my life. We are all energy and vibration. I can believe and think about what I wish. The price I pay is my vibration. I check in with myself by asking, *What I am THINKING*. I know that what I think about, I bring about. If it is not positive, I throw it away. I thought I could temporarily revisit my prior pattern of negative complaining and then easily return back to my positive statements. Big lessons. I was a yoyo for years, going back and forth, doing positive prayer and then waking up negative. My vibration will attract from the viewpoint of my perception.

Today, I can deliver unconditional love, by embodying spiritual principles, such as acceptance. I did not know how to do this before. I no longer have a victim perspective. I play a part. We are on earth for a short time. I believe in live and let live. I send love and acceptance to wherever all beings are at on their journey. We all have a journey. I was given my journey to allow others to learn in theirs. Enjoying the process of unfolding is the most delicious part.

I invest time, energy, and money in my own well-being today. This is a self-esteem action for me. I must take care of me. I prioritize and ask myself how I feel. This is the most important. Prioritize and the Universe will shift as to the vibration I exhibit. One of the original barometers that I learned early on and still use is HALT. Don't get too Hungry, Angry, Lonely or Tired. I monitor this daily. If I don't feel right, I ask myself why I feel the tension. Is something off? Do I feel overwhelmed? Am I hungry? When is the last time I ate something? Am I cranky? Am I tired? Am I lonely? Do I need to call someone? Do I have a form of self-pity? Do I feel resentment? I self-evaluate or ask another for feedback.

Upon awakening every morning, before I do anything, I honor God (Source) (insert name) for a minimum of twelve minutes. I honor our connection together. It's my devotional. If I get up on the wrong side of the bed, I start my day over. I can do this at any time during the day, and it has been necessary if I do not feel right. When I feel separate from my Creator, I must ask myself, "Who moved?"

After forty years, the self-talk has changed. Today I know the Truth. I see the truth. I speak the truth. I have discovered that I am divinely protected, even when so-called *bad things* happen. I feel connected to the greater good. I have more peace of mind. I no longer feel like I am going it alone. When I focus on God, Spirit, the eye of the storm, and Christ within me, wherever I focus is where I am headed. When I focus at this moment on what is real and true, I align with my true self and experience joy, peace, and contentment. I ask. I listen. I focus on thoughts aligned with my Creator's view of me. I allow my vibration to rise. It works if I work it. It is amazing how healing works. It's an inside job with an inside answer.

All spiritual and religious healers have been of extraordinary help to me. I have been told by more than one advisor, counselor, and healer that I have experienced more traumas in one lifetime than any one person could ever handle. Taking chemicals was my reaction to my understanding of what was happening to me as a child within the alcoholism environment and to help me feel better. Did I step on the toes of others and suffer from their retaliation? Yes, in an arrested development process. I re-experienced trauma and felt powerless at the time. I sought professional help once again in 2016 and new layers of healing began again.I could see my part and moved to self forgiveness and forgiveness of others.

Today, I do not feel any powerlessness. It is gone. I am no longer traumatized. I closed the door to the perpetrators. I took care of me. No matter what the circumstances, my vision, and the steps are up and forward at every turn. My needs are met. God has equipped me with a roof over my head, a nice car to drive warm meals to eat. I am eternally grateful.

I would like to pretend I know everything, but this is part of false pride. What I do know is that using any kind of chemical, or covering up, or running is never the answer to truth and healing. Real healing is being able to look and deal with the dark side, the demons, and asked to release them, so my true light could enter.

Many layers later the white light is all that remains now. I am free. I am free to acknowledge the disease of perception—*and as I shift my perception and change my thoughts, I am free to be the beautifully-made me.* One of the greatest gifts in my journey is discovering my purpose: I am here to bring hope, joy, and inspiration and to deliver this information to you. This is my vehicle to be of service.

*Until you make the unconscious conscious, it will
direct your life, and you will call it fate."*

— CARL JUNG

CORONAVIRUS COVID-19

In December 2019, the city of Wuhan in Huber Province China. The seventh largest city comprising 11 million residents became the center of Pneumonia outbreak of unknown cause, with global implications. The Chinese health authorities conducted an immediate investigation of these clustered cases to identify and control its spread by isolating suspected infected patients, closely monitoring their contracts and obtaining detailed clinical and epidemiologic data.

In early January 2020, Chinese scientists isolated a novel coronavirus (CoV) from the patient groups in Wuhan. The outbreak is believed to have started at a local seafood, wild animal market. As of February 11, 2020, is officially known as severe acute respiratory syndrome (SARS) coronavirus 2 *SARS-CoV-2 the novel virus that causes coronavirus disease 2019 (COVID-19) reference.medscape.com.

Over these last weeks all businesses are shut down. Millions upon Millions of people filing unemployment. I am self-employed and I for the last 22 years depended on face to face contact. I am out of a job. I have no income until I decide to generate something else for myself and or the virus is controlled. From my humanitarian perspective, I know this is necessary and as a person who has overcome alcoholism and drug addictions, I realize just how difficult this time is for those wanting or have a desire to stop drinking or using and have nowhere to go for help. Face to face contact is an absolute necessity for an addicted individual. It is his/her lifeblood. Due to our social restrictions during this time it is recommended to stay away from other people. This too shall pass. There is telephone help for recovery meetings for those wanting sobriety or those attempting to maintain sobriety. Telephone meetings are growing in population thanks to our internet carriers. Also, those with cancer, heart disease has their own challenges. I hope and pray all who need help will receive help, even modified help such as the telephone, internet, zoom, at this time in our world. This is a very challenging time and a time for all people to open their hearts and help one another where ever possible. Taking one minute to place a telephone call, a snail mail letter or an email.

The pandemic happened I believe because the world and people in our world were divisive. I am sad for our lives lost. We have experienced powerlessness. Our divine power, our creator wanted the world to come together and one the major ways to come together is for all individuals to have a common bond. It seems our world lesson is we needed to come together. To unite as one. This may be an answer to prayer. The event seems like we are forced to isolate however, this is only physical isolation. Right now All the human minds in the world must unite. We must stay united for a good stretch of time. Our nations are sharing information to help one another. Let's keep our principles of unconditional love while we stay put and continue to help ourselves and our neighbors.

A MESSAGE OF HELP FROM DR. ROBIN TO YOU

There is a way. If I can overcome one hundred plus obstacles in my lifetime, you can too. If I can make it, I absolutely know you can too. If you feel overwhelmed, as I did, and want to give up, don't. I will pray for you and hold the knowledge for your healing until you can know it for yourself. I love and am here to bring joy, inspiration, and happiness to those who not only need it as well as ask for it.

As a result of my journey of recovery and healing, I came to see that these are true—*and can be true for you:*

- I have received more than one God shot (blessing) in my life.
- Even when I was mistreated or betrayed, the blessing was still in my life, though I could not see it, touch, or feel it.
- None can come against what Spirit has blessed, and the blessing causes me to stand up.
- Someone may have hurt me or betrayed me, but they did not stop my destiny.
- The blessing is more powerful than the curse.
- When people ignore me and try to push me down, it will cause me to be noticed.
- The good breaks will find me.
- I don't have to convince people to like me.
- I can erase my social media history and message.
- I don't need people's approval
- People may have not kept their word, but my intention is I keep my word.
- Like Jacob from the Bible. I keep doing the right thing. I keep being the best I can be.
- I remain teachable and stay encouraged by removing my illusionary limits of Spirit's power.
- My gifts and talent can change from being ignored or slandered to being favored.
- Folks can see me in a new light. They can come to respect me.
- I must enlarge my vision, not shrink it. I feel the vision.

- My dream may look impossible, but "with God, all things are possible."
- Everything is always working out for me, though I may not see it yet.
- Generational blessings are coming my way.
- The abundance of my blessings cannot be contained.

I am available for Speaking, Spiritual Coaching,
Energy Alignment & Acupuncture Services at:

949-568-0776

12340 Seal Beach Blvd Suite B-195 Seal Beach, Ca 90740

Afterword

Emmet Fox states, "There is no God we meet.... only consciousness." We transcend or change form, and our physical body is discarded. When we expire, we keep our energy body, and our energy bodies move back to our energetic plane. Chinese Medicine teaches that our corporeal soul, which is housed in the lung, stays with our body and our ethereal soul, Hun (PO) moves on. I now see the energetic bodies that exist. They are light-bodied. I see them throughout my house. I know that I have a spirit guide, and I see him. I was born with it. We are all born with it. If we improve our vibration for a few minutes a day, over time, we can use our senses to communicate, to receive and send. We must be able to tune into the vibrational frequency, like tuning into a desired radio station. All of us are operating at different levels of frequency. We become more connected to the unseen energies if we operate at a higher frequency. To receive, we must tune into, create and feel the higher frequencies.

The Taoists refer to the "Wu Qi," commonly translated as the infinite, to describe a base state of undifferentiated oneness, from which the duality of yin and yang emerge, to separate further into "the myriad," or the millions, the material, or shared reality, that makes up our physical existence. This similar concept is defined in quantum physics as the "zero-point field," or the field of infinite potential, or the field of all possibilities. This is the field that fills the spaces in-between. It is the place we can access through higher vibrations, assisted by conscious intent to shift patterns of information that manifest both physically and non-physically.

"Most folks are as happy as they make up their minds to be."

— **ABRAHAM LINCOLN**

I used to be upset because I wanted—*and thought I needed*—someone or something to help me feel better. I was relying on some outer fix. My happiness has everything to do with me. To help me with that, I can perceive life from a viewpoint of *this moment in front of me* and then put each moment together for twenty-four hours. One day at a time. Life is only this place, this time, and these people, right here and now. This I can handle.

"What you are looking for, you are looking with."

The twenty-four-hour principle also applies to my looking at what I am emitting into the Universe. My output is important. What I am expressing in energy, thought, word and action make a difference in how I feel. I feel my way into my dream, vision the picture of my dream, set the goals to allow the dream to materialize, express the energy, thoughts, words, and actions of those goals, and let the dream manifest. I manifest what I emit. One important caveat: When I plan out my goal, I do not attach myself to when, how, or where the outcome will occur, or what it will look like. I leave this up to a greater force than I, _ _ _a Higher Power, who lies deep within.

"Change your thinking, change your life."

"If it is to be, it is up to me."

I finally understood what my mom was conveying to me. *I love you, mom.*

About the Author

Dr. Robin Roemer-Brown is a California State Board Certified Acupuncturist, Diplomate of the National Commission for the Certification of Acupuncturists in 2000. She is a graduate of the University of California, at Santa Barbara, South Baylo University and received professional training from Beijing, China in 1994 at California location and 1998 in Bejing. In 1997 she was licensed by the State of California Board of Medical Quality Assurance. Dr. Robin Roemer Brown is a former associated Professor of Oriental Medicine. She received training at the Beijing Academy of Traditional Chinese Medicine and Traumatology at Wang Jing Hospital in China. Dr. Robin received the Top Doctor Awards for Worldwide Leaders in Healthcare in the International Association of Healthcare Professionals in 2018 and is an honored member of Continental Who's Who.

Since 1997, Robin Roemer-Brown specializes in helping immune disorders and those with symptoms of low libido, fatigue, cold hands, feet, loose stool, low back pain, hypothyroidism type symptoms. Robin worked with pain managment for 20 years and has been a recovery advocate for 40+ years.

Robin Roemer-Brown's background encompasses American and Oriental Herbology, Diagnostic Muscle Testing for Applied Clinical Nutrition, sports medicine, athletic training, (she was, in fact, a World Amateur Triathlete/Biathlete champion in 1989-90 earning 87 road racing trophies and awards) Mental Health and Spiritual Training as well as a diversity of other healing arts. She uses a whole-body approach combined with integrative West-to-East medicine techniques. Dr. Robin also works as a consultant and is able to help make positive changes in people's lives by helping them to see themselves, walk-in balance and improve homeostasis utilizing dietary and lifestyle advice. Dr. Robin uses a wealth of knowledge and training, she became a licensed minister 12-12-2012, Dr. Robin operates as a *spiritual advisor* utilizing fortune telling, palm, pulse reading, offering body, mind and spirit assistance. She is currently a consultant online and is available to speak.

Dr. Robin Roemer Brown can be reached at 12340 Seal Beach Blvd Suite B 195, Seal Beach, CA 90740. Call 949-568-0776.

* 9 7 9 8 5 3 7 1 6 6 5 4 2 *